Successful Professional Portfolios for Nursing Students

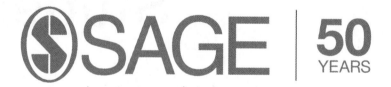

SAGE was founded in 1965 by Sara Miller McCune to support the dissemination of usable knowledge by publishing innovative and high-quality research and teaching content. Today, we publish more than 750 journals, including those of more than 300 learned societies, more than 800 new books per year, and a growing range of library products including archives, data, case studies, reports, conference highlights, and video. SAGE remains majority-owned by our founder, and after Sara's lifetime will become owned by a charitable trust that secures our continued independence.

Los Angeles | London | Washington DC | New Delhi | Singapore | Boston

2nd Edition

Successful Professional Portfolios for Nursing Students

Suzanne Reed

$SAGE | **m** LearningMatters

Los Angeles | London | New Delhi
Singapore | Washington DC | Boston

KH

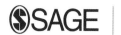

Learning Matters
An imprint of SAGE Publications Ltd
1 Oliver's Yard
55 City Road
London EC1Y 1SP

SAGE Publications Inc.
2455 Teller Road
Thousand Oaks, California 91320

SAGE Publications India Pvt Ltd
B 1/I 1 Mohan Cooperative Industrial Area
Mathura Road
New Delhi 110 044

SAGE Publications Asia-Pacific Pte Ltd
3 Church Street
#10-04 Samsung Hub
Singapore 049483

Editor: Alex Clabburn
Production editor: Chris Marke
Copy-editor: Diana Chambers
Proofreader: Sue Edwards
Marketing Manager: Camille Richmond
Cover Design: Wendy Scott
Typeset by: C&M Digitals (P) Ltd, Chennai, India
Printed by: Henry Ling Limited at The Dorset Press,
Dorchester, DT1 1HD

© Suzanne Reed 2015

First published 2011
Second edition 2015

Library of Congress Control Number: 2015932452

British Library Cataloguing in Publication data

A catalogue record for this book is available from
the British Library

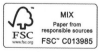

MIX
Paper from
responsible sources
FSC
www.fsc.org   FSC™ C013985

ISBN 978-1-4739-1631-9 (pbk)
ISBN 978-1-4739-1630-2(hbk)

5/9/16

Contents

Transforming Nursing Practice is a series tailor-made for pre-registration student nurses. Each book in the series is:

- ○ Affordable
- ○ Mapped to the NMC Standards and Essential Skills Clusters
- ○ Full of active learning features
- ○ Focused on applying theory to practice

Each book addresses a core topic and they have been carefully developed to be simple to use, quick to read and written in clear language.

> An invaluable series of books that explicitly relates to the NMC standards. Each book cover a different topic that students need to explore in order to develop into a qualified nurse... I would recommend this series to all Pre-Registration nursing students whatever their field or year of study
>
> **Linda Robson**
> **Senior Lecturer, Edge Hill University**
>
> The set of books is an excellent resource for students. The series is small, easily portable and valuable. I use the whole set on a regular basis.
>
> **Fiona Davies**
> **Senior Nurse Lecturer, University of Derby**
>
> I recommend the SAGE/Learning Matters series to all my students as they are relevant and concise. Please keep up the good work.
>
> **Thomas Beary**
> **Senior Lecturer in Mental Health Nursing, University of Hertfordshire**

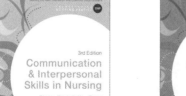

3rd Edition
Communication & Interpersonal Skills in Nursing
Shirley Bach & Alec Grant

2nd Edition
Patient Assessment and Care Planning in Nursing
Lioba Howatson-Jones, Mooi Standing & Susan Roberts

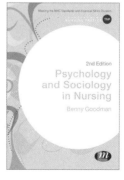

2nd Edition
Psychology and Sociology in Nursing
Benny Goodman

ABOUT THE SERIES EDITORS

Professor Shirley Bach is Head of the School of Health Sciences at the University of Brighton and responsible for the core knowledge titles. Previously she was head of post-graduate studies and has developed curriculum for undergraduate and pre-registration courses in a variety of subject domains.

Dr Mooi Standing is an Independent Academic Consultant (UK and International) and responsible for the personal and professional learning skills titles. She is an accredited NMC Quality Assurance Reviewer of educational programmes and a Professional Regulator Panellist on the NMC Practice Committee.

Sandra Walker is Senior Teaching Fellow in Mental Health at the University of Southampton and responsible for the mental health nursing titles. She is a Qualified Mental Health Nurse with a wide range of clinical experience spanning more than 20 years.

CORE KNOWLEDGE TITLES:

Becoming a Registered Nurse: Making the Transition to Practice

Communication and Interpersonal Skills in Nursing (3rd Ed)

Contexts of Contemporary Nursing (2nd Ed)

Getting into Nursing (2nd Ed)

Health Promotion and Public Health for Nursing Students (2nd Ed)

Introduction to Medicines Management in Nursing

Law and Professional Issues in Nursing (3rd Ed)

Leadership, Management and Team Working in Nursing (2nd Ed)

Learning Skills for Nursing Students

Medicines Management in Children's Nursing

Nursing and Collaborative Practice (2nd Ed)

Nursing and Mental Health Care

Nursing in Partnership with Patients and Carers

Passing Calculations Tests for Nursing Students (3rd Ed)

Palliative and End of Life Care in Nursing

Patient Assessment and Care Planning in Nursing (2nd Ed)

Patient and Carer Participation in Nursing

Patient Safety and Managing Risk in Nursing

Psychology and Sociology in Nursing (2nd Ed)

Successful Practice Learning for Nursing Students (2nd Ed)

Understanding Ethics in Nursing Practice

Using Health Policy in Nursing

What is Nursing? Exploring Theory and Practice (3rd Ed)

PERSONAL AND PROFESSIONAL LEARNING SKILLS TITLES:

Clinical Judgement and Decision Making for Nursing Students (2nd Ed)

Critical Thinking and Writing for Nursing Students (2nd Ed)

Evidence-based Practice in Nursing (2nd Ed)

Information Skills for Nursing Students

Reflective Practice in Nursing (2nd Ed)

Succeeding in Essays, Exams & OSCEs for Nursing Students

Succeeding in Literature Reviews and Research Project Plans for Nursing Students (2nd Ed)

Successful Professional Portfolios for Nursing Students (2nd Ed)

Understanding Research for Nursing Students (2nd Ed)

MENTAL HEALTH NURSING TITLES:

Assessment and Decision Making in Mental Health Nursing

Engagement and Therapeutic Communication in Mental Health Nursing

Medicines Management in Mental Health Nursing

Mental Health Law in Nursing

Physical Healthcare and Promotion in Mental Health Nursing

Psychosocial Interventions in Mental Health Nursing

ADULT NURSING TITLES:

Acute and Critical Care in Adult Nursing

Caring for Older People in Nursing

Medicines Management in Adult Nursing

Nursing Adults with Long Term Conditions

Safeguarding Adults in Nursing Practice

Dementia Care in Nursing

You can find more information on each of these titles and our other learning resources at **www.sagepub.co.uk**. Many of these titles are also available in various e-book formats, please visit our website for more information.

Foreword to the first edition

In the increasingly litigious world of healthcare there are important lessons for nurses to learn in order to avoid subsequent court room or NMC disciplinary hearing appearances. Shortcomings in nurses' record keeping is the second most common category of hearing brought before the nursing and midwifery regulator. This compact new textbook is a timely addition to the nursing literature in offering nursing student readers an opportunity to embark on a journey that will sustain them throughout the whole of their professional lives. The journey alluded to here is the process of keeping and maintaining a professional portfolio.

In this book, readers are offered tangible, clear and unambiguous instruction on building and maintaining a sustainable professional portfolio. All nursing students are cognisant of the need to ensure that their record keeping is meticulous. They all understand that they have a professional and legal duty to keep records which are clear, intelligible and accurate. Hence, NMC policy is clear in highlighting the importance of nurses making records which are accurate and recorded in a way that ensures the meaning is clear. The discipline of keeping and maintaining a professional portfolio has been highlighted by the NMC as an aid to developing these skills.

Portfolio keeping as a discipline is advisable as it acts as a concrete focus for reflection in both learning and clinical environments. The evident link between keeping a portfolio and reflection offers the individual student a lifelong approach to dealing with the everyday complexities of life as a nurse in contemporary healthcare settings. The discipline of keeping a professional portfolio has many benefits for the individual embarking on the journey, not least being the ability to recall through the pages of the portfolio events which may have happened years before.

Each of the seven chapters in this book is designed to depict, through examples, the benefits of keeping a professional portfolio harnessed to reflection. The recording of one's own feelings on how an individual decision was made and how it relates to the personal lived experience of being a nurse is what makes this book so special.

Linking your own career with the keeping of a portfolio not only makes good sense but is likely to impress future employers, all of whom take portfolio keeping very seriously as the epitome of professional nursing. Suzanne Reed has designed and written a book which I commend to you as an essential acquisition to ensure the viability of your transition from nursing student to registered nurse and beyond.

Professor Edward Alan Glasper
Professor of Nursing
The University of Southampton

About the author

Suzanne Reed is an experienced General Manager with many years working at strategic and operational levels in the NHS and independent sector. Senior posts held include Ward Manager in medicine and neurology, Director of Academic Affairs and Associate Dean for the development and assessment of pre- and post-registration nursing and midwifery programmes, Head of Department, and General Manager for clinical quality and multidisciplinary education. Suzanne was an accredited reviewer for the approval of NMC nursing preparation programmes and a managing reviewer for quality monitoring of NMC nursing, midwifery and health-visiting programmes. Currently, Suzanne is a freelance writer and a voluntary carer in the community. Awards include winner of the Sister Dora Silver Medal for clinical practice and a Florence Nightingale Scholarship to study clinical assessment in Canada. Suzanne has been a key speaker at many international and national nursing conferences, and has published many articles in refereed journals as well as a nursing textbook on evidence-based practice.

Contributor

Alison Clark is a Lecturer in the School of Nursing, Midwifery and Physiotherapy at the University of Nottingham. She teaches across nursing theory and practice with a specific remit for public health and health promotion, and also teaches health psychology, professional development and mentorship. She has implemented learning sets to support practice-based learning for mentors and students, and has developed practice-led portfolios and web-based resources for mentorship, securing funding from two Centre for Teaching and Learning Excellence sites. Alison continues to work with a local cancer support group to maintain her interest in the psychosocial care of people with cancer and their carers.

Acknowledgements

Throughout the time it took to write this book, life went on. I would like to thank my husband who encourages me in everything I do, making it possible for me to maintain focus on the things that matter.

This book would have been so much less without the abundance of talent and contributions from Alison Clark and students from the University of Nottingham School of Nursing. I would also like to thank Professor Edward Alan Glasper for sharing his knowledge and providing numerous tips. Finally, a big thank you to Richenda Milton-Daws who read my drafts and helped me to say what I wanted to say, fixing my errors and advising on sections that needed rewriting for clarity.

Suzanne Reed

Introduction

Keeping a portfolio is an important part of your preparation for nursing. It encourages you to reflect both on your learning in the lecture room and on your experience in the clinical arena, and in this way to gain the maximum benefit from both. It also ensures that you have a written record of your preparation programme. This will give you something to refer to when you need to refresh your memory, and also means that you have evidence to show to tutors, examiners and (in time) prospective employers. Eventually, your portfolio will feature as an essential requirement of revalidation with the NMC and your self-development for fitness to practise.

What does this book cover?

The idea of compiling a portfolio can seem overwhelming at first. This book sets out to demystify the process, and give clear and friendly guidelines for getting started and keeping going. It also demonstrates the long-term benefits of portfolios, both for your own learning and self-development, and to enhance your career prospects.

Chapter 1 looks at what a portfolio actually is and the importance of reflection for portfolio writing, describes the 6Cs for nursing (DH, 2012) and related behaviours, and suggests how you might get started on putting together a portfolio. This chapter introduces you to four students from different fields of practice who are all approaching this task for the first time.

Chapter 2 is concerned with professional development planning and how making a personal development plan contributes to an effective portfolio.

Chapter 3 looks at what other evidence you should be collecting to put in your portfolio and how to distinguish between different types of evidence. This chapter also shows how the 6Cs for Nursing can be applied to clinical practice.

Chapter 4 looks at ways of presenting your evidence and introduces the idea of keeping a portfolio in electronic format. This contributes to a discussion on using your portfolio specifically to demonstrate your achievement. Chapter 5 examines another major use of your portfolio – as a reflective record of your learning and one that can enhance your learning experience throughout your course.

Chapters 6 and 7 look forward to the end of your preparation programme and beyond. Chapter 6 is concerned with how an effective portfolio can be used for assessment, while Chapter 7 looks at how a continuing portfolio can help you to set career goals and demonstrate your competence at all stages of your professional life, and how to use your portfolio as part of the NMC revalidation process. A great advantage of reading this chapter while you are still a nursing student is that it really shows you how your three-year preparation programme relates to the career you will have after you qualify.

NMC *Standards for Pre-registration Nursing Education*, essential skills clusters and the 6Cs

The Nursing and Midwifery Council (NMC) has standards of competence that have to be met by applicants to different parts of the nursing and midwifery register. These standards are what the NMC deems as necessary for the delivery of safe, effective nursing practice. As well as specific competencies, the NMC identifies specific skills that nursing students must have at various points of their training programme. These essential skills clusters (ESCs) are essential abilities that students need to attain in order to practise to their full potential.

Compassion in Practice (DH, 2012) describes nursing as an extraordinary role which has deep significance, providing care for people from the joy at the beginning of a new life to sadness at its end. Our work is conducted in a wide variety of settings, supporting people in our care and their families when they are at their most vulnerable. Our work presents us with challenges and occasionally you may encounter care which falls short of what people have a right to expect. We all have a professional commitment to tackle these challenges, and you must never underestimate your significance or the capacity you have to make a difference and ensure that people are cared for with dignity, respect and compassion. Six types of behaviour representing fundamental nursing values, features and characteristics have been identified (DH, 2012), which are at the heart of everything that nurses and other healthcare staff do in the course of their everyday work. These types of behaviour all begin with the letter C and have come to be known as the 6Cs. The 6Cs each carry equal weighting.

- Caring – is the core business of nurses.
- Compassion – is based on empathy, dignity and respect, and how care is delivered.
- Competence – is the ability to understand health and social care needs, and having technical and clinical expertise to deliver evidence-based care.
- Communication – is central to teamwork; listening to patients is as important as what we say and do.
- Courage – is speaking up when we have concerns, and ensuring that the patient's voice is heard and acted upon.
- Commitment – is following through with actions to solve issues and improve the patient's experience.

This book identifies some of the competencies and skills that student nurses need to be able to demonstrate in order to be entered on to the NMC register. These competencies are presented at the start of each chapter so that it is clear which of them the chapter addresses. All of the competencies and ESCs in this book relate to the generic standards that all nursing students must achieve. The 6Cs will also be referred to throughout the text.

Activities

At various stages within each chapter there are points at which you can break to undertake activities. Undertaking and understanding the activities is an important element of your understanding of the content of each chapter. You are encouraged, where appropriate, to reflect on your practice and consider how the things you have learned from working with patients might inform your understanding of exactly what nursing is. Other activities will require you to take time away from the book to find out new information that will add to your understanding of the topic under discussion. Some activities challenge you to apply your learning to a question or scenario to help you reflect on issues and practice in more depth. A few activities require you to make observations during your day-to-day life or in the clinical setting. All these activities are designed to increase your understanding of the topics under discussion and how they reflect on nursing practice. The emphasis is always on how to record your experience and reflections in such a way as to deepen and demonstrate your learning.

There is a short glossary of terms at the end of the book which you may find useful. Glossary terms are in **bold type** on their first appearance.

Chapter 1
What is a portfolio?

NMC Standards for Pre-registration Nursing Education

This chapter will address the following competencies:

Domain 1: Professional values

7. All nurses must be responsible and accountable for keeping their knowledge and skills up to date through continuing professional development. They must aim to improve their performance and enhance the safety and quality of care through evaluation, supervision and appraisal.
8. All nurses must practise independently, recognising the limits of their competence and knowledge. They must reflect on these limits and seek advice from, or refer to, other professionals where necessary.

Domain 2: Communication and interpersonal skills

7. All nurses must maintain accurate, clear and complete records, including the use of electronic formats, using appropriate and plain language.

Chapter aims

After reading this chapter you will be able to:

- understand why reflection is important for compiling a portfolio;
- identify with a range of materials you might collect as evidence of professional and personal development (learning);
- consider how best to organise and present your portfolio;
- define a portfolio, and explain what yours means to you.

Introduction

Portfolios are often used in pre-registration **nursing** programmes to demonstrate and assess learning. It is therefore important that you have the direction, guidance and skills necessary to collate one successfully. Many pre-registration nursing students feel quite bewildered about what a portfolio is and what they should keep in it. This can lead to anxiety and a sense of being overwhelmed; not knowing where to begin and what to do (Timmins and Dunne, 2009; McMullan, 2008). This chapter will give you some insight into how to produce a successful portfolio, where to begin, what to include and, most importantly, how to 'showcase' your learning. This will be built on in later chapters.

Much of the work needed to put a portfolio together involves reflecting on your experiences, both in the classroom and on placement, and considering carefully what you can learn from them. If you use reflection in this way, the portfolio becomes an ongoing learning tool as well as a way of demonstrating your achievements. You will find more about reflection, and in particular about keeping a reflective journal as part of your portfolio, in Chapter 3.

In this chapter, four pre-registration nursing students – Aimee, Jeff, Alex and Natasha (all pseudonyms) – share their early experiences of compiling their portfolios and how they managed to overcome some of the challenges:

- understanding what a portfolio is and its value in demonstrating learning;
- working out what should go into it and why;
- ensuring that they get into the habit of reflecting upon experiences, rather than simply recording them;
- beginning to plan and organise a portfolio;
- comparing the merits of an e-portfolio against the merits of traditional, paper-based portfolios.

What is a portfolio and how can it demonstrate your learning?

Your portfolio will be a collection of carefully selected materials which provide a snapshot of your student journey from the beginning of your pre-registration programme to successful completion, and eventually beyond registration. As an accessible resource, its value will be in how well it reflects and verifies your current, recent and past learning experiences and activities. The materials are usually collated in a hard-backed ring binder for easy access. Some students, however, now keep electronic versions known as e-portfolios, and although you will need to keep to either an electronic or a paper copy for when you present your portfolio for assessment, you may well find it helpful to use both electronic and paper folders for your own purposes.

If you have just started your nursing preparation programme, you may feel you do not have anything to go into your portfolio. You do, though! You will be able to bring learning from school, from your hobbies or voluntary work, or from previous work experience. Once you start to reflect on what you have learned from these, you will find you have already absorbed plenty of skills and knowledge which will be useful in becoming a nurse.

Activity 1.1   *Reflection*

To ensure that the NHS has a culture of caring and putting patients first, all nursing course applicants are now tested on their values (Latham, 2014). It is also a requirement that students spend some time working in a care capacity to gain prior experience to confirm they are certain they want to be a nurse. Think back to your application and interview for nursing. What life experiences did you claim had already given you some insight into what being a nurse meant and the skills required to work with people?

Working out what goes into your portfolio and why

You may have done voluntary work with people with learning disabilities, perhaps taken them on holiday; or managed staff in an office; or helped put on a school play; even brought up a family. These kinds of activities and work experience will bring with them a range of interpersonal and communication skills which are essential for good nursing; for example, you may have developed sound organisational and time-management skills in balancing part-time work with study. You may be surprised to find that these attributes are all relevant to the NMC's four domains for nursing practice (NMC, 2010c) which you will be working to develop during your nursing programme. In addition, many schools of nursing will ask you to undertake some kind of self-assessment activity to identify your learning needs. Your personal academic record may include some exercises related to self-assessment of certain study and learning skills (see Chapter 2). Read the case study below to see what life experience each of our four pre-registration students has that might be relevant to nursing and how they identified their learning needs with their personal teacher.

Case study

Aimee has just left sixth-form college. During her work on the college newsletter she interviewed staff and students about current events which were influencing the school. In her spare time she has worked with Mencap, taking children with learning disabilities on holiday. She wants to work with people with learning disabilities.

Jeff has just completed his BTEC in health and social care at the local community college. He left school at 16 and went to work in a local supermarket where he has worked for the last four years. He plays football at the weekends and lives with his partner Jane in a flat in the city. He hopes to become a mental health nurse.

Alex is 31 years old and he has had several jobs (working as a mechanic). He is married with two children, both at school, and acts as a school governor. He has taken three A levels at night school over

continued ...

continued ...

the last two years. He is interested in working with children who have long-term illnesses when he qualifies.

Natasha is 45 and worked in IT, after gaining her degree in computer studies. She decided she needed a career change and chose to become a nurse, working within the adult field of nursing. She has four grown-up children who all now live away from home. She has elderly parents, one of whom requires 24-hour care due to a long-standing illness.

The first column in Table 1.1 lists the kinds of material (content) that can go into a portfolio. The rest show how all four students were able to demonstrate that they have valuable life experience which they can bring with them into their nursing course. Their personal tutor then helped them to profile their past experiences and complete a reflective assessment of their current strengths in dealing with people, how they might organise their time around work and home life, and what their specific learning needs might be. This is sometimes known as a SWOT analysis, that is to say, you identify where you feel your strengths are, where you feel you need to develop (weaknesses), how you might develop (opportunities for) and what might hinder your learning (threats). This will be addressed in more detail in Chapter 2.

All four students felt confident about their ability to communicate with people. Aimee, Jeff and Alex all felt fairly confident with their study skills and organising a balanced home and work life. Natasha, however, expressed some concern about how she would manage her home, work and parental caring responsibilities. She felt it would be really important to be well organised and schedule in her commitments in order not to feel overwhelmed. She felt she had the skills to do this even though it was some time since she had done formal study. Jeff and Alex were more concerned about working within a team of highly trained professionals and how they would fit in, especially Alex who, as a more mature student, was worried that a lot more would be expected of him as he was older. He felt vulnerable as, while he was happy to look after and work with well children, nursing sick children would be a whole new experience for him. (Natasha echoed Alex's concerns about how she would be seen as a mature student.) Aimee was looking forward to the challenge of working with more disabled children, but worried about how she would 'cope' with working in more institutionalised settings.

Activity 1.2   *Critical thinking*

Aimee, Jeff, Alex and Natasha were able to consider how to put together their portfolio with the help of their personal teacher. Referring to the simple list of **evidence** in the first column of Table 1.1, have you any similar materials that you have already collected and popped in a box file somewhere for safe keeping? Sort through them. Think about what they say about you, how they show your current strengths, attributes and areas for development. Organise them into relevant sections for your portfolio.

Potential portfolio content	Aimee	Jeff	Alex	Natasha
A curriculum vitae (CV) work history				
Personal/educational development certificates	A-level Biology, English Literature and French	BTEC in Health and Social Care	A-level Biology, Physics and Chemistry	BSC Computer Sciences A-level History, English and Art
Work-based training courses	IT/media training on newsletter	Health and safety Food hygiene	Health and safety School governor training	IT training Ergonomic safety Equality and diversity training
Self-assessments: • ways in which you prefer to learn; • initial SWOT analysis and personal. development/action plan	Personal statement in application	Personal statement in application BTEC portfolio	Personal statement in application Learning styles inventory for foundation study skills	Personal statement in application Vocational guidance counselling
Assessment from others: • references • testimonials	Personal statement from Mencap holiday manager First aid certificate	References: • work • BTEC (seen)	References: • work • college • school governor	References: • work • volunteer work organiser (hospice)

Potential portfolio content	Aimee	Jeff	Alex	Natasha
Evidence of learning from life or work experience: 1. Diary/journal extract 2. Feedback from others: • thank you cards • accounts of community/ professional activities professional professional activities	Raising money for local charity Thank you card from children and parents Sample newsletter from sixth-form college	Being captain of the football team – planning and organisation notes	Summary of school governor activities	Summary of working as volunteer doing gardening at local respite/hospice centre
Ongoing SWOT and personal development/action plans	SWOT Study skills OK Good communicator – face-to-face and written Managed to work with people with learning disabilities but worried about working in more institutional setting with severely disabled	SWOT Study skills OK Good communicator and managed people Needs academic support (dyslexia)	SWOT Study skills OK Good communicator and can take a lead in a group Older, so will people expect more?	SWOT Study skills OK Good communicator, strong IT skills Led a team Managing father alongside course – worry Older, so will people expect more?

Table 1.1: What could go into a portfolio?

At this stage don't worry if you have collected only a few materials – you will soon see it grow. Start saving any materials and documents which you think reflect your learning. One way to start is to make notes from what you are learning in your classroom sessions, or from any related practice activities. Note down your thoughts and feelings, and any factors you think were influencing your learning, as well as what you think you learnt in each situation. These records might be useful for later reflection (see Chapter 3).

Using reflection

Get into the habit of reflecting on your experiences. A useful strategy for making key notes to reflect on how much you are learning is to ask yourself the following three questions.

1. What have we been doing in class today?
2. What have I learnt?
3. Why will this be important when I come to actually providing nursing care to people? (Clark, 2010a, 2010b).

Case study

Alex did this exercise. He came out of a session on child development thoroughly confused by all the different theories the lecturer had skimmed over. He spent an hour putting his notes together and real-ised that if he didn't understand some aspects of child development he may not understand how illness can influence normal child development, or the relationship between brothers and sisters, or even how well a parent may bond with their child if it is born with a health problem or disability. He realised how important this was in being able to empathise with families of ill children and perhaps in being non-judgemental in the way he approaches families. Alex also realised that if he did the same exercise when he was on placement, he might be able to link the nursing care he was seeing back to some of the theory he was being taught in the classroom.

Your portfolio provides one means of helping you to consider the application of classroom learning and how this links to your clinical skills. For example, you may have spent time in class considering nursing models and the nursing process, and been told this links to how patient care is planned and implemented. This will not seem real, perhaps, or relevant until you *see* nurses working with patients and their carers in planning, giving and documenting their care. You may also find other ways that 'care planning' is described, such as 'care pathways' or 'care packages', and come to realise that underpinning each is a systematic approach to nursing people (i.e. the nursing process). Alternatively, you may see nurses working to improve current practice, the patient experience, the information provided to patients and carers, and the way services are organised to meet patients' needs. In doing so, nurses are actively informing the way we as nurses work in the future.

How to use your portfolio to demonstrate compassionate care

The strategy document *Compassion in Practice* (DH, 2012) identifies six different types of behaviour which represent features and characteristics of everything that all nurses do irrespective of which field of nursing you work in. You will see that the features and characteristics all begin with the letter C so they have come to be known as the 6Cs. The 6Cs are at the heart of how nurses work in practice and they have implications for what you are taught during your programme and for what you do throughout your nursing career. Each of the 6Cs carries equal weighting; they are:

- caring;
- compassion;
- competence;
- communication;
- courage;
- commitment.

The following matrix explains what is involved in each of the 6Cs. The left side of the matrix shows features and characteristics of the 6Cs and the right side describes related values and behaviours.

Features and characteristics of the 6Cs	Values and behaviours related to the 6Cs
Care is the core business of nurses. The patient is viewed as the priority. Effective care improves the health of individuals and communities	Patient-centred care is assessed, planned, delivered and evaluated Nurse involves the patient in decisions about their care
Compassion is how care is delivered through good relationships between nurses, patients and relatives	Nurse is empathic, treats patients with dignity, humanity, respect and kindness
Competence is having the ability and knowledge required to deliver effective high-quality evidence-based care	Nurse has up-to-date clinical knowledge and skills, technical skills and research awareness Identifies risk and prevents harm to others
Communication is about effective teamwork The ability to speak clearly to patients and relatives Provides reassurance to patients and relatives	Nurse has good listening skills, reporting and recording skills, has rapport with patients, relatives and colleagues, is approachable

(Continued)

(Continued)

Features and characteristics of the 6Cs	Values and behaviours related to the 6Cs
Courage is speaking up when the nurse has concerns Seeks out feedback	Nurse has integrity and ethical values Shows accountability
Commitment is taking action to improve the patient and relative's experience, increasing transparency	Nurse is open and responsive and creates a positive and safe culture Candour, honesty

(Based on Watterson, 2013)

Activity 1.3   *Critical thinking*

Using the above matrix, write a short script describing the behaviours which would be helpful in comforting a friend who is going through a tough time. Search for things you might do no matter how small they may seem, which may reassure and support your friend. File the script in your portfolio under a section headed the 6Cs.

The Nursing and Midwifery Council Code of Conduct

In 2015 the NMC approved a new professional code for registrants (NMC, 2015). The new code is centred around four topics – prioritising people, practising effectively, preserving safety and promoting professionalism. Key instructions included in the new Code of Conduct reaffirm the importance of the 6Cs. It is intended that the new code will be a live document used to address good practice, leadership and using all forms of communication responsibly. The new code features instructions designed to help you treat people with compassion and to ensure that their physical, social and psychological needs are assessed and met. There will also be information about exercising candour when errors or harm occur. Your portfolio will be a valuable tool that you can use to demonstrate good practice that follows the NMC Code of Conduct.

Beginning to plan and organise your portfolio

The NMC (2010c) views portfolio compilation as an important part of a nursing programme and suggests that portfolios:

- provide a means for negotiating, directing and affirming learning;
- facilitate self-directed, individualised learning;
- 'showcase' ongoing development, personally and professionally, which can be used formatively and/or summatively to assess progress against predetermined criteria (and gain academic credit as well as verification of achievement of practice competencies);

- help integrate theory with practice and practice with theory (even to the extent of developing the theory that informs nurses' practice);

- develop the skills of reflection and critical analysis;

- provide an opportunity to express learning in more creative ways other than the usual written notes and reflections on and about nursing practice (Timmins and Dunne, 2009).

Your **ongoing achievement record (OAR)** and your clinical assessment document which you will keep in your portfolio will follow you from one placement to the next (discussed further in Chapter 3); each **mentor**, as well as your personal teacher, will be able to see at a glance where you are progressing in terms of your programme and clinical competence assessments. One option for keeping your portfolio will be within a ring binder, with neatly divided sections for relevant material. However, some of you will be asked, or maybe choose, to keep an e-portfolio.

Comparing the merits of e-portfolios and traditional paper-based portfolios

E-portfolios have increasingly replaced traditional paper-based methods of storing evidence in a ring binder. Studies have shown that many students prefer this to paper formats. Research by Strivens et al. (2009) suggests that e-portfolios might provide information that is more related to how you learn, as well as what you learn. That is to say, the *rich and complex processes of planning, synthesising, sharing, discussing, reflecting, giving, receiving and responding to feedback* which are essential skills in enhancing learning (Strivens et al., 2009, p9). E-portfolios can also make it easier to include electronic materials, making links to information that you have accessed to inform your practice (anything from YouTube to a database to a patient forum). In addition, you might want to include photographs, audio and video files (provided you follow the usual rules about consent, anonymity and **confidentiality** where they are related to actual patients and staff). Finnerty et al. (2008) suggest that for e-portfolios to work well you will need to ensure that you have clear goals for your learning; guidelines on the type of evidence you will need to provide to prove your learning; relevant and accessible IT support; and a willingness to engage with your tutor, and possibly fellow students, regularly (as some e-portfolio work can be through discussion forums). Table 1.2 illustrates some of the perceived benefits of e-portfolios as expressed by students and their tutors.

Efficiency	Enhances learning
Work all in one place	IT skills enhanced
Less likely to be lost	Flag a learning event/reflect later/focuses thinking
Mobile	Process of learning can be seen as well as outcome
Accessible 24/7	Track progress easier

(Continued)

Table 1.2 (Continued)

Efficiency	Enhances learning
Early help if gaps in progress seen	Tutor feedback more quickly available
Allows for input from several sources	Creativity in selection of evidence
Pre-set structure enhances organisation	Helps planning/organising learning
Gives a time framework for learning (history)	Easier to link evidence
Easier to access	Reflection on value of evidence enhanced
Allows reader to 'jump' quickly between parts	Assists in self-assessment
Easier to link evidence	Presentation skills for different audiences
Interactive and collaborative	

Table 1.2: Perceived benefits of an e-portfolio (adapted from Strivens et al., 2009 and Finnerty et al., 2008)

It is important, regardless of the type of portfolio you maintain, that all of the contents in your portfolio are kept confidential. So always keep in mind who it is for, who will be looking at it and who will have access to it. Any details (of patient, family, practitioner or trust) must be anonymised. It is also important that you have a sense of owning your work and feel you can decide some aspects of its content, what goes where and when.

Activity 1.4   *Critical thinking*

Consider the value of a portfolio as noted by the students in this chapter. Then, think about what your portfolio means to you, what benefit it will be to you in your pre-registration programme and throughout your nursing career.

Complete this statement: My portfolio will be ....

To summarise, a portfolio says something about you, your life and work experiences, and more particularly what you have *learnt* from them, your known strengths and areas for development. It's an ongoing process.

Throughout your nursing programme you will need to show your personal and professional development through working with a range of people with health and social care needs, and working within multidisciplinary teams and across health and social care agencies.

Defining a portfolio

Your portfolio will provide evidence of some of your learning. It will follow you from one practice learning experience to the next. Each mentor, as well as your personal teacher, will be able to see where you are in relation to your developing competence (your growing knowledge base, developing a range of practical, technical and interpersonal skills, and becoming increasingly professional in your approach to clients).

Activity 1.5   *Critical thinking*

Read the following definition of 'what a portfolio is' and, using your own words, sum up what you want your portfolio to reflect about you, and your personal and professional development.

Contemporary portfolios can be viewed as having many functions for both qualified and undergraduate nursing students preparing for professional practice. (Timmins, 2009)

There is no answer provided for this as you must make your own decision about what a portfolio can do for you, and its value in reflecting some of your learning.

There are distinct differences in the way we describe the purpose and value of portfolios. In the first, it is seen as 'end product' of your learning activities and experiences: a means to show you can link the theory you learn in school with practice experiences and vice versa. Each placement will offer you different learning opportunities and your mentor(s) will help you sum up your learning against achievement of the required NMC competencies in your ongoing achievement record, and then a continuation for maintaining and updating skills and knowledge following initial registration. The second, however, emphasises more the learning process – that of critical reflection on and about the practice you will both see and participate in with mentors and other healthcare professionals. **Critical thinking** and **reflection** are explored more fully in Chapter 3; however, the following two definitions introduce a simple description about the importance of both terms.

- Critical thinking *engages our reasoning as we ponder theories, arguments and debates. A competent nurse is one who selects the relevant information to plan a course of action and then judges what is best to do in a given circumstance. The nurse has to be competent in managing risk.* (Price and Harrington, 2013, pp2, 3)

- Reflection is a way of examining your experience in order to look for the possibility of other explanations and alternative approaches to doing things. It may happen as an activity or when you have more time to think about what you have experienced. (Howatson-Jones, 2013, p15)

- Scholes and her colleagues (2004) emphasise reflection as a learning process but add the need to be able to initiate your own learning. The role of the mentor is seen as that of an assessor, making a judgement about the extent of your progress. This can be an area of conflict of interest for your mentor. While they will have your interests at heart in facilitating your learning, and providing educational and clinical support, they must also act as a 'final judge' in verifying your learning at specific stages of your nursing programme. So a portfolio can have a dual function: it can say something about how you go about your learning and what you have learnt, for personal and professional development, to direct and affirm it. However, portfolios can also be used as a means to verify learning. What and how you select material to include in your portfolio is therefore important. Some people can go about this in a very hap-hazard way, collecting material which they think shows their learning and then making sense of it later (see Figure 1.1). However, a more useful way to set about compiling a portfolio is to start with some idea of what you want to learn, and why (see Chapter 2 for more details).

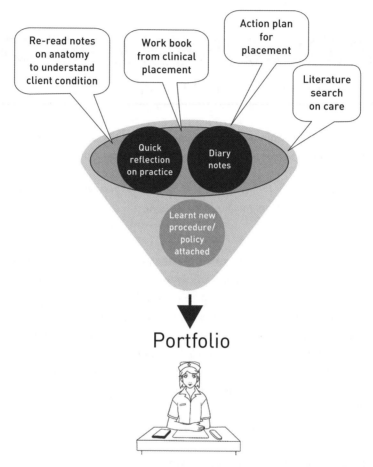

Figure 1.1: Now how do I make sense of all this?

Activity 1.6   *Reflection*

Which one are you?

Style 1

You have decided to go shopping with a friend. You're not sure what you need, but it will be nice to go and have a look around. If you see something nice you might buy it. You have £25.00 left in your purse and take your credit card just in case you need more.

continued ...

continued ...

Style 2

You decide to shop with a friend. You make a list of the things you need and know how much you can afford to spend. You have £25.00 in your purse and can use your debit card for a further £10.00 if you need it.

You will probably be familiar with both styles of shopping. How many times have you come home with things you didn't expect to buy, or realise you already have the same item in your wardrobe, or more tins of beans than you can manage in the next month? How many times have you come home without the much needed item? If you are to avoid unnecessary loss of time and undue expense it's better to have a plan. The same goes for compiling a portfolio. Students often present with lots of information they have collected while they have been in practice but when they come to look at it again its meaning and value has been lost. You need a plan. The next section looks at how our four students planned to start their portfolio.

Getting started on your portfolio

Aimee, Jeff, Alex and Natasha are about to start their first practice learning experience. In order to show they are developing personally and professionally they will need to add to the portfolio materials they put together from their interviews and preparation for the course. They can do this in several ways as follows.

1. Make a list of their expectations, fears and concerns to discuss with their tutors.
2. Make a personal development or action plan for their practice experience.
3. Plan what material they will collect to show what they have learnt from their first semester, including for example:
   - record the initial visit to the practice learning environment and meet their mentor;
   - record an exercise to look up a specific type of nursing, or a particular client need in the library or on the web (see Chapter 2);
   - make notes from shadowing the patient's journey, e.g. observing investigative procedures, attending out-patients, working alongside other health professionals such as physiotherapists, speech therapists, dieticians and occupational therapists, or reports and documents from project work;
   - written evidence of learning experience in the classroom and from clinical placements;
   - written summaries or reports from any practice-based project work, e.g. analysing how to use the most appropriate health education materials for clients;
   - mind maps to show awareness of the different roles of healthcare professionals and/or agencies in supporting clients' health and social care needs;

- feedback from others in the form of witness statements or testimonials, thank you cards, annotations in their ongoing assessment records, appraisals from personal, or module, tutors and feedback from assignments and projects;

- poems, stories and paintings can also be used to demonstrate learning (see Chapter 3).

4. Written reflection on various aspects of their experience during the first semester:

- ideas from students who have been working there before (with some caution as not all students will gain from the same placement in the same way);

- annotated, anonymised patient care documents, which will help to show how they have worked with clients and/or their family members, or with other healthcare professionals;

- reflective diary excerpts/notes about care experience – for example, about coming to understand why notions of stereotyping and stigma were explored in class and seeing how they become relevant when working with specific patient groups;

- reflective writing around a client and their care needs, for example understanding informed consent, or what factors limit patient choice or concordance with treatment.

The above are only examples of the range of materials that the four students could select to begin to build their portfolios. What is important to remember is that your portfolio needs to reflect your learning (not what you have done), and that it can be a part of your assessment of your progress throughout your programme.

Case study: Getting started

Aimee, Jeff, Alex and Natasha each worked with their personal tutor to decide what materials they could collect to show their learning. None of them was sure which materials would be 'the best' for showing their learning and why. They were worried about how to interpret the competencies within their evidence. Their personal tutor talked them through the pros and cons of each form of evidence, explaining that while they needed some evidence that reflected self-assessment of their progress, this needed to be balanced by feedback from their mentors and other healthcare professionals. In addition, it would be good for them to show that they were 'studying' nursing by making connections between the taught theory in school and practice and vice versa. They need to show that they are not only learning to nurse but also learning to think critically about why they are nursing or caring for clients in a particular way or using specific approaches to meet care needs (see Chapters 2 and 3).

The students realised that an action plan, identifying what they want to learn from their placement, may help them decide what kind of evidence to collect with their mentors. (There is more about types of evidence in Chapter 3.) Their mentors would then also have a baseline from which to plan and add appropriate learning opportunities. They decided to:

- *arrange a visit to their placement;*
- *formulate a personal development (action) plan, setting out individual learning needs and possible ways to achieve them (an action plan) to discuss with their mentors (see Chapter 2);*

continued ...

continued …

- *keep a diary on care activities;*
- *reflect on learning experiences in the classroom and how they might apply to their clinical placements;*
- *gather personal statements from experts and mentors to demonstrate their progression;*
- *collect a range of annotated, anonymised patient care documents to demonstrate their thoughts about and rationale for practice.*

Aimee and Alex's first placement was working in the community. Their aim was to know more about 'the lived experience' of people with a learning disability and mental health problems, and that of their families. They wanted to know what and who was there to help them. They thought reflective writing and making notes on shadowing other healthcare professionals in order to understand their role would be useful ways to show how much they had learnt about their clients' needs, who met them and how.

Jeff and Natasha, on the other hand, were both working in acute care settings. They were concerned about developing their clinical care skills with clients who were acutely ill. They felt that they were likely to be working in a very busy care setting with little time for in-depth reflection. They felt they would rather keep a 'nursing notes diary' and then follow up with some reflection at a later stage to help them understand the implications of their experiences.

All the students realised that they had different things they wanted to learn. In focusing on collecting two types of evidence, which would support the direct observation from their mentors, they would also be able to become skilled in formulating particular kinds of evidence. They had a plan on which to focus their learning and work, and from which to expand.

A plan for your portfolio can be useful as a basis for directing, focusing and verifying your learning activities with your mentor. Your mentor will arrange a series of meetings with you (usually at least two formal ones at the beginning and end of your placement; preferably three if it's a longer placement), bringing their mentoring experience to provide an interim review of your progress. At these meetings you will want to plan further learning, refining your plan if you were overoptimistic regarding what it was possible to learn in the time and with the resources you had available. Your mentor will make an overall judgement of your progress from their own observations and those of others (see Chapter 4). Your personal tutor will also discuss your progress at regular intervals and discuss how that is reflected in your portfolio, as well as by your overall performance in the course (usually at the beginning and end of each semester). In addition, portfolios are sampled by external examiners to affirm and validate the assessment strategy in your school. The quality of the material in your portfolio is therefore of the utmost importance.

You need to:

1. plan and direct your own learning, initially with the support of your mentor and tutor;
2. pick up on opportunistic learning that has added to your experience;
3. make sense of your learning by reflecting on and critically thinking about your practice in a variety of ways;

4. record your progress against the NMC competencies, as well as your own aims for learning;

5. be clear on the criteria being used for assessment of your portfolio work (see Chapter 4).

Activity 1.7   *Decision making*

Referring to the simple list of evidence created by Aimee and Alex in Table 1.1, identify any similar materials and documents you have collected so far. Sort through them, organise them and insert them in your ring binder or in the relevant sections of your e-portfolio in a way that they reflect your learning to this point in your course.

If you are at an early stage you will have only collected a few materials to insert in your portfolio but don't worry, you will soon see it grow. However, if you are further on into your course you may want to consider the types of evidence you have collected so far, how well they reflect your progress, and if there are different types of evidence that might add to your portfolio which would broaden and deepen how well it demonstrates your professional development from semester to semester, or over the last year of your course.

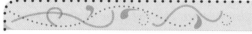

Chapter summary

This chapter has looked at what a portfolio is and why it is helpful to compile one. It draws a distinction between simply listing experiences and achievements (although this is useful to indicate to superiors and prospective employers what you have done) and reflecting upon them. Reflection about an experience or event deepens your understanding of its significance and therefore your learning. The chapter has considered exactly what you should be including in a portfolio and why, and gives some initial advice on how to get started.

Further reading

Clark, AC (2010a) How to compile a professional portfolio of practice 1: aims and learning outcomes. *Nursing Times,*106 (41): 12–14.

Clark, AC (2010b) How to compile a professional portfolio of practice 2: structure and building evidence. *Nursing Times,* 106 (42): 14–18.
Both of the above provide a useful outline for organising a portfolio.

Department of Health (DH) (2012) *Compassion in Practice.* London: HMSO.
Sets out the new strategy for nursing and defines the 6Cs.

Howatson-Jones, L (2013) *Reflective Practice in Nursing* (2nd edition). London: SAGE Publications.
Gives a comprehensive account of reflection and benefits to an individual, workforce and to patient care.

Latham, D (2014) Test for nursing values unveiled. *Nursing Times*, 22 October, 10 (3).

Describes the new system for assessing the values of applicants to nursing courses and potentially those qualified staff applying for new posts.

Lintern, S (2014) Prior experience for students is the bottom line. CNO Summit, Lord Willis. *Nursing Times*, 110 (51).

Provides the reasons for prior experience before embarking on a career in nursing. Informs of the likely change from a previous report of one year prior experience to less time.

Price, B and Harrington, A (2013) *Critical Thinking and Writing for Nursing Students* (2nd edition). London: SAGE Publications.

Provides the context of critical thinking and separates the different connotations through several meanings.

Read, C (2014) More work to do to make the 6Cs universal. Report of the CNO for England Summit 2014. *Nursing Times*, special edition, 110 (50).

Describes the important work needed to embed the 6Cs into everyday practice.

Buykx, P, Kinsman, L, Cooper, S, McConnell-Henry, T, Cant, R, Endacott, R and Scholes, J (2011) Educating nurses to identify patient deterioration: a theory based model for best practice simulation education. *Nurse Education Today*, 31 (7): 687–93.

The learner moves through phases of experiencing, reflecting and thinking through the reflective process.

Watterson, L (2013) 6Cs + Principles = Care. *Nursing Standard*, 27 (46): 24–5.

Looks at the relationship between the 6Cs and principles of nursing practice.

Useful websites

http://standards.nmc-uk.org/pages/welcome.aspx

The Nursing and Midwifery Council (standards page) provides information about the new *Standards for Pre-registration Nursing Education* and the essential skills clusters (published autumn 2010), which should be referred to in your portfolio.

Chapter 2
Personal development planning

Chapter aims

After reading this chapter you will be able to:

- discuss the merits of planned and opportunistic learning, and how each can be represented in your portfolio effectively;
- understand how a personal development (action) plan can guide your learning;
- complete a SWOT analysis and a rudimentary action plan to guide your learning around a given area of practice.

Introduction

In Chapter 1 we explored the merits of keeping a portfolio. A **personal development plan (PDP)** is a key part of your portfolio. It will provide a framework for you to identify your strengths and help you plan your learning where there are areas needing development. You will not, however, be aware of how much there is to learn, what is essential to learn, what might be nice to learn and what to learn, when. This is where your mentor, or personal tutor, will be able to identify possible learning opportunities for you. Also, you will encounter learning experiences from patient care situations that could not have been planned for or anticipated by you or others. If your portfolio is to successfully demonstrate your learning, you need to capture both the planned and the unexpected.

When you have thought about your personal development plan, you need to think again about what you put in your portfolio.

Your personal development plan

The PDP is a structured and supported process, undertaken by a learner to reflect upon their own learning, performance and/or achievement and to plan for their personal, educational and career development. (QAA for Higher Education, 2009, pp2, 5)

In nursing, the PDP will help you identify specific, focused pieces of learning which will reflect your developing patient care management skills; for example, communicating with distressed people, educating people to manage their medicines, ensuring infection control or understanding anatomy, physiology and pathophysiology; ways to assess and approach meeting clients' needs; and developing your skills to work in a multidisciplinary setting. Your PDP will have value because it will set your personal learning goals, thoughts and ideas against those predetermined by your nursing programme and the NMC competencies. Your plan will also enable you to review your progress on an ongoing basis, and identify appropriate steps to remedy any gaps in your learning, by yourself, or with your mentor or personal tutor.

There is a variety of approaches to personal development planning. The University of Salford's Faculty of Health and Social Care has published a *Personal Development Planning Resources Pack* (2007, p8), which indicates five stages to producing a personal development plan:

1. self-assess;
2. plan;
3. do;
4. review;
5. record.

Much of your learning will be driven by your experiences in the classroom and in practice settings as you proceed through your course. Figure 2.1 (overleaf) shows how Kolb's (1984) experiential cycle of learning can be adapted to offer a five-stage model which incorporates personal development planning. In addition, you may find that your university has its own guidelines and activities which will help you.

Alternatively, in order to focus and create your own personal development plan you may like to follow these six steps:

1. identify an aspect of patient care you want (need) to learn;
2. assess your current learning needs;
3. plan for the learning you need to do;
4. decide on the best method or approach that will help your learning;
5. record your learning;
6. evaluate your learning.

In each of these two schemes, the steps to personal development planning are similar. However, in the one recommended in this text, making a decision about the learning methods you might use to achieve your PDP (step 4) has been added as this may influence your learning. In addition, the sixth step, evaluating your learning, mirrors the way in which, in the figure, the arrow sends you back to the beginning of the cycle, ensuring that you monitor and measure your learning (not just record it) and recommence the cycle to ensure ongoing learning.

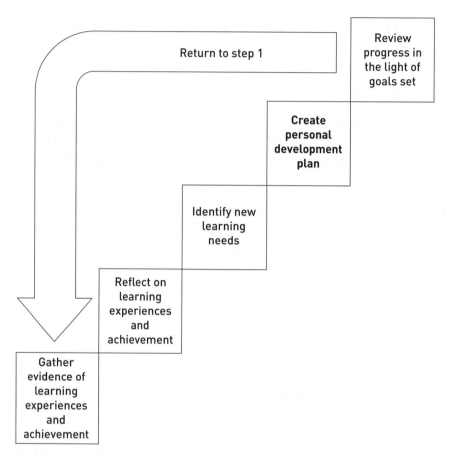

Figure 2.1: Personal development planning: the five-stage cycle of effective learning
(Source: based on the ideas of Kolb, 1984)

Did you notice that steps 1–4 also closely link to the self-assessment technique known as the SWOT analysis referred to in Chapter 1? This is the first stage in drawing up your PDP; the second is planning your learning (steps 3–5); and the final one is summing up how much you have learnt and how much you still have to learn.

The following section takes you through each stage in more detail. On its completion you will be able to complete a PDP, around one or more aspects of nursing practice, to share and refine with your tutor or your mentor. The example of 'doing the drugs' is used to illustrate how to identify the knowledge, skills and professional issues that you will need to consider and build upon during your practice experience (for the full essential skills criteria, please see the list of useful websites on page 21).

Step 1: Identify an aspect of patient care you want or need to learn

The easiest and most effective way to identify what you need to learn, and to what extent, is to look at one or more of the following:

- module learning outcomes;
- the competencies and essential skills clusters;
- the student learning package for your practice area;
- local and national guidelines, procedures and protocols for best practice.

At this stage it may be useful to focus on one or two small aspects of your module learning outcomes. For instance, this might be in understanding the link between learning anatomy and physiology and pharmacology, and how that influences your clinical skills development.

The NMC (2007b) has decided that 'doing the drugs' requires you to:

- be numerate, so you can calculate dosages of commonly used medication (see 4.1 of the field standard for competence for children's nurses and ESC 33);
- be able to administer drugs to the patient correctly (six Rs; see box below), with full knowledge of the purpose of the medication, its usual dosages, possible side-effects and contraindications (under direct supervision);
- recognise when the giving of a drug may be inappropriate;
- recognise when adverse reactions occur and act appropriately;
- assess and monitor patients who give their own drugs (self-administration);
- know what action to take if errors occur and act accordingly;
- work within current legislations regarding the storage, transport, prescription, administration and disposal of drugs;
- work within a multiprofessional team to ensure medication is appropriate and safe for patients, e.g. doctors and pharmacists;
- understand your accountability for safe drug administration when working in different care settings, e.g. the patient's home.

In relation to 'doing the drugs', the first progression point (end of first year) only asks you to be able to show that you can calculate commonly used drug dosages safely and know the process for administering drugs under supervision (see Figure 2.2, steps 1–4 in particular).

Six Rs for the administration of medicines

- right person;
- right drug;
- right date and time;
- right dose;
- right route;
- right prescription.

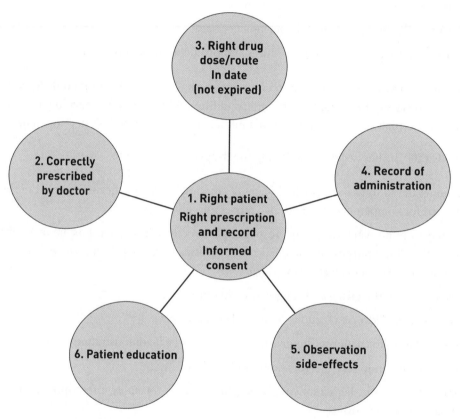

Figure 2.2: 'Doing the drugs'

(Source: based on NMC, 2007b)

The greater responsibility for understanding how the drugs work, monitoring the patient's reaction to the medication, and working with the doctors and pharmacists is left to your mentor while you 'get the basics'. However, as you progress your mentors will expect you to be aware of how legislation affects who can prescribe and give drugs to patients, when and how, and eventually to work with the patient and other healthcare professionals. As you will be formally assessed on your ability to 'do the drugs' some time within your field-related programme, it is important to plan your learning, taking small steps to achieve the whole competence.

Step 2: Assessing your current learning needs

Consider the following to help you to decide where to focus your learning activities.

What do you need to learn now for your portfolio?

- Identify your strengths; where do you feel confident or competent?
- Look for any gaps (weaknesses) in your knowledge base, your skill and/or approach to managing this aspect of patient care.
- What do you feel you need to improve now? What can be left until later?

Activity 2.1 *Reflection*

Re-read the NMC requirements for 'being safe' in drug administration. Now use the following continuum to assess the degree to which you feel confident and competent to 'do the drugs' with your mentor, safely, in relation to each criterion.

I feel very confident (score 10 if you are at this end of the scale)	←——————→	I do not feel at all confident (score 1 if you are at this end of the scale)
I think I am very competent (score 10 if you are at this end of the scale)	←——————→	I still have aspects to learn to be competent (score 1 if you are at this end of the scale)

Clark (2010b) has found this a useful way of helping students during their practice experiences to self-assess where they are in relation to developing specific nursing skills and their underpinning knowledge, and to plan further learning. You will see through later discussion how four second-year student nurses' personal development plans reflected how they each had different learning needs to address in relation to achieving the desired progression points.

Step 3: Plan the learning you need to do

It is useful to have specific things you want to know and to decide how you will measure your progress (and what evidence you will collect for your portolio).

Some people find it helpful to write aims and objectives to guide their learning, and to identify what would help them learn, and what evidence they would collect to verify their progress with their mentor or personal tutor. A useful acronym for this is SMART. This stands for specific objectives, which are measurable, achievable, realistic and timely.

So while you might aim to become more confident and competent in managing patients' medications, you will need goals that are:

specific – clear goals such as 'practise calculations', 'practise giving medication by different routes' and 'observe and learn how mentors teach patients about their medication', that can be easily ...

measured – through observation by and discussion with your mentor, and reflections on working with patients and/or their carers to ensure they understand their medication. You will also need to ensure your goals are ...

achievable – i.e. that there will be sufficient medicines administered to patients for you to observe and practise under supervision by your mentor – and ...

realistic – i.e. your goals must be obtainable within the practice learning environment – and ...

timely – while you are in placement, with opportunities for complementary study while you are in university.

You also need to know what support mechanisms are available to help you achieve your aim, including e-learning resources, textbooks and help from your fellow students, and even sometimes from the patients.

To sum up, steps 1–4 help you do a 'SWOT'. Working in this way means you will be less likely to feel overwhelmed by how much there is to learn or disheartened if you don't manage to achieve it all.

Using a SWOT in practice

Ask yourself the following three questions.

- What do I want/need to learn?
- What will help me learn it?
- How will I know I have learnt it?

Case study

Joanne and Mike are both second-year nursing students. Joanne is a learning disabilities nursing student and Mike is a children's nursing student. One of the aims of their shared module on pharmacology was 'to understand the nurse's role in medicine management'. They both felt a little overwhelmed when they realised that this included understanding how drugs work, drug side-effects

continued ...

continued ...

and interactions; local Trust policy and legislation; the procedure for drug administration; and how to provide health education to patients and their carers. They were also aware that they had a 'drug administration test' to undertake some time over the next four placements (ESCs). Mike felt he could easily learn some of the more factual elements around how drugs work in relation to the children he would be nursing. His main concern was in 'doing the drugs', and being able to calculate medications safely, particularly for babies. Joanne was more concerned about how people with learning disability problems could manage their own medication, and how to teach them to self-medicate. They shared their SWOT analysis with Samina and Tim. Samina (a mental health student) had seen a lot in the press about mental health patients' medication being monitored and supervised. She was interested in learning more about factors that influence whether patients with mental health problems took their drugs or not, and most of all what she would do if a patient refused their medication. Tim (adult nursing) was happy preparing for the actual essential skills assessment on drug administration as he had already had lots of practice in his clinical placements. He was more worried about what would happen if he made an error. He didn't feel too confident either about approaching doctors or pharmacists if he had concerns about a patient's medication or their prescription. Between them they recognised that there was a lot more to 'doing the drugs' than they had previously realised. They discussed what was important for them to learn in their next placement and what could possibly be left until later on when they had more experience (see Mike and Joanne's SWOT analysis in Table 2.1). All four students felt more confident to discuss what they wanted to learn with their mentor.

Mike		Joanne	
Strengths	**Weaknesses**	**Strengths**	**Weaknesses**
Good numeracy skills because I achieved a high grade in my maths exams I passed year one's maths test Know the six Rs, have read hospital policy and NMC guidelines	Still find calculation of drugs for children, especially babies, scary. Lots of drugs seem to come in syrups and lotions rather than pills – still not sure how this affects 'adding up' and dosage calculations Not had to give a child an injection yet Not had to help parents understand medication	Have watched and assisted mentors and carers with drug management on community placement = six Rs Realise what happens if drugs not given on time or not given with/ after food Know not to crush drugs for those with enteral feeds	Not sure about how people with learning disabilities can learn about their medication and self-medicate What legislation and protocols are there to follow or techniques for teaching self-management Still not confident about my maths, so how will LD patients cope?

continued ...

Mike		Joanne	
Opportunities	**Threats to learning**	**Opportunities**	**Threats to learning**
Next placement surgical ward ... 'do the drugs'/ practise drug calculation under supervison (might practise a lot and save the ESC test until third year)	Busy five-day ward, my mentor won't have time to spend with me to practise Time – other assignments and ESCs to do What happens if I make an error? – anxious	Next placement assessment unit Find the protocols See if there is any literature on self-medication and learning disabilities Watch how staff help people learn to manage own medications	Clients likely to have poor communication/ cognitive skills which will hinder ability to self-medicate – so might not see new patient being taught self-medication
Opportunities	**Threats to learning**	**Opportunities**	**Threats to learning**
Ward's link lecturer or pharmacist might give me some sample calculations Seen a 'drug calculations for nurses' textbook that might be useful – use library or buy one Review NMC and Trust guidelines		Find out if clients have specially prepared medications so no drug calculations needed Redo maths test for practice prior to placement See support teacher	Fear if I tell someone something wrong Time

Table 2.1: Mike and Joanne's SWOT analysis

In completing their SWOT analysis the four students had identified some possible learning opportunities to discuss with their mentors and refined their action plans. They had answered the following five questions.

- What are my learning needs?
- What challenges might I encounter?
- What adjustments might I need to make?

- Who are the key people who can help me in the university and while I am on placement?
- What are my goals and priorities?

Activity 2.2　　　　　　　　　　　　　　　*Reflection and decision making*

Pick an aspect of your nursing practice you want to develop. You could do this around 'doing the drugs' and compare your learning needs to Mike's and Joanne's.

Assess your learning needs by using a SWOT analysis exercise and the questions above (or any other strategy you might find on the internet or in your university study skills web pages). Remember to refer back to the module outcomes, competencies and essential skills for ideas about the breadth of knowledge and skills you need to develop.

Make a provisional plan for future learning to discuss with your mentor and personal tutor.

You will probably have realised that being a nurse means you are constantly learning. You need to be able to prioritise what is important to learn now; what can be built on through your learning experiences; and what can be learnt later (put on a 'back burner', so to speak) until you have the important fundamental knowledge and skills within your grasp. The next step is to consider how you learn best and how other people can help you learn.

Step 4: Decide your best method of learning

The next step is to decide the best method to achieve your learning. It has been suggested by several educationalists that this will depend on your preferred **learning style**. Learning styles are various approaches and ways of learning that are presumed to enable you to learn best. It is believed that most people favour a particular style which can help to direct the methods of teaching and learning that suit you best. The most widely used system for assessing learning styles is that of Honey and Mumford (2000) who developed the work of Kolb (1984). Honey and Mumford identified four types of learning styles: activist, reflector, theorist and pragmatist. These styles are not fixed and can be changed at will or by circumstance. A short simple explanation of each style and corresponding relevant learning method is given below (adapted from reviews by Frankel, 2009; Clark, 2008; Mobbs, 2003; Honey and Mumford, 2000).

Activists like to be involved in new experiences (mindset: 'will try anything once'), are open-minded and seek challenges, but get bored easily. Their preferred ways of learning are trial and error, actual practice (hands-on), simulations of practice, undertaking case studies, problem-solving activities, small group discussions, role play, puzzles and competitions. They tend to like being thrown in at the deep end to learn and find themselves acting as chair-people in meetings or leading discussions. They don't like reading, writing or thinking on their own, lectures, or having to follow instructions to the letter. Downside: they tend to act first and consider the consequences later, and like to be the centre of activities.

Reflectors prefer learning methods where they can gather data and information, ponder on it, analyse facts and then act. They tend to be thoughtful and listen to others before offering their own views. Mindset: tend towards the cautious. They prefer to be thoroughly briefed about their practice before they do it; plus use reflective learning logs or journals to debrief on and review events; find mind mapping or concept mapping useful techniques; like self-analysis question- naires, paired discussions, observing activities and problem-based learning. They are people who listen, reflect and then contribute. They don't like to work to tight deadlines, being thrown in at the deep end, taking a lead on role-playing activities. Downside: they have a tendency to take a back seat and appear distant.

Theorists like to think things through, are rational, and reject subjectivity and flippancy. They like things to be logical. These people learn through lectures, seminars and analogies, which help them understand the complexities of nursing practice; they like to be convinced that what they are learning is important, relevant and up to date; they like structure and to have a clear purpose in learning. They like discussion groups which facilitate more thorough debate of theories and application to practice. They don't like unstructured teaching events or ones where emotions and feelings are emphasised as part of the outcomes. Downside: they tend to be perfectionists.

Pragmatists prefer searching out new ideas and putting things into practice. They like problem-solving activities and making decisions quickly. (Mindset: there is always a better way.) They need to understand the relevance of the learning activity; like observing experts and then doing nursing; and like working in skills laboratories to 'practise first', case studies, role play and field work. They respond well to coaching and feedback – role models are important to them. They like teaching others what they have learnt. They learn less well when there is no obvious benefit to them, when no guidelines are available and when it seems to be 'all theory'. Downside: they have a tendency to be impatient with long drawn-out discussions (they like to get on with things).

At a glance, do you fit into any particular style of learning? You will probably find that whereas one style may describe the dominant way you learn, you already adopt different ways of learning depending on the circumstances. Mike discovered his learning style was that of an activist – he likes hands-on practice. This style fits with his plan to do the drugs and calculations time and again to prepare for his assessment and fit his learning around his experiences. Joanne found that she was more suited to a reflective learning style. She wants to make sure that she under- stands the theory and policy behind self-medication before learning how to assess patients' ability to self-medicate.

This is only the briefest of introductions to learning styles. There are many different ways of determining your learning style. It is beyond the scope of this book to give detailed guidance on finding out your learning style, and your university is likely to offer exercises to help you explore ways you learn. Talk to your tutor if you need further guidance on finding out your learning style, or refer to the Further reading and Useful website suggestions at the end of this chapter.

Activity 2.3   *Research and finding out*

Using one of the published tools available, identify your dominant learning style. Note down the corresponding, relevant learning methods from the list above that would most suit your style. Think about any ways you might need to develop your study methods to be more effective in learning about nursing and doing nursing (note there may be a cost to this exercise as you may need to pay to access the tools).

How you learn is important; your learning style is only one factor to consider. A useful guide to learning in the workplace can be found at the Campaign for Learning (**www.campaign-for-learning. org.uk**). This website offers more tips on how to think about and organise your learning. The final stage of the personal plan development process, however, is summarising your overall learning, documenting it, verification and looking to future learning needs (restarting the personal development planning process).

Step 5: Recording your learning

By now you will have drafted some realistic aims for learning, and identified some opportunities for and ways of learning. This next step involves how you record your learning experiences in relation to achievement of the NMC competencies, and showing the link between practice and theory. This will need to be a concise, comprehensive record of what has happened in the course of your learning process and the outcome. The four students worked alongside their mentors and other staff, and achieved most of their goals on their action plan. Their mentors verified their learning from a range of opportunities that occurred while on their placements. In Mike's case, even though his mentor was very busy, she ensured he had lots of practice 'doing the drugs' with other trained nurses on the ward. Mike made regular diary notes of the children's medications, how they worked and where he had to calculate dosages. He also managed to complete two informal (formative) practice assessments with one of the other staff nurses in preparation for later assessment on drug administration. He was also able to show a reflection he had completed on teaching a parent about ensuring their child complete a course of antibiotics post-surgery (see the summary of his personal development planning, Table 2.2). Joanne was able to show her mentor how she had worked consistently with one adult with a learning disability on how to manage his daily medication. She presented her case study with appendices to show her reading around the topic, and that she understood local and national policy on self-medication. Both students were able to record this in their ongoing assessment records.

Step 1	Step 2	Step 3	Step 4	Step 5	Step 6
Identified module learning outcomes/ clinical outcomes related to medication management	SWOT analysis – concern Calculation of drugs in common use for children Increased awareness of the importance of competence in drug calculation – babies Not given injection yet Not liaised with medics and pharmacists (later objective perhaps)	My priority – to be more competent in calculation of drugs in common use with children, especially babies Do the drugs as much as possible, prep for ESC Practise under supervision of mentor in placement – 1:1 giving drugs to one child and explain medication to parent	Select suitable activity/method of learning Shadow mentor on drug rounds Do common calculations at least once a week Talk to pharmacist, mentor and expert nurses, personal teacher	I worked out a reasonable timeframe and how I would record the learning I achieved Date my competencies achieved Evidence submitted – diary notes, reflection	Completed learning activities and collected evidence which was verified by my mentor and tutor Learning summary in my portfolio New action plan for next placement Do a group of patients' medicines Liaise with pharmacist and doctors more Find out about responsibilities for ordering, transport, storage of meds – next placement community so might be more important

Table 2.2: A summary of Mike's simple personal development plan

Building in unplanned learning opportunities

Consider building some degree of flexibility into your PDP to allow for extra time in the event of changes or unforeseen events. It is not always possible to anticipate learning experiences or opportunities that may come along during your practice experience. A useful way to maximise learning from the business of your everyday working experiences as a student nurse is to ask yourself the following three questions.

- What have I done today?
- What have I learnt today?
- What do I need to learn next?

You could do this by reflecting on the care activities you have been undertaking, on a patient situation or on a professional issue that has arisen.

Case study

Samina, the mental health student nurse, had been working in an elderly mentally infirm unit. Many of the patients had various forms of dementia. They needed a lot of support physically, socially and psychologically. There wasn't a lot of time left in the working day for her to sit down and reflect on her practice. Her tutor had popped in to see her on placement and Samina expressed her frustration at not getting time to do 'proper reflection' on her practice. Her tutor suggested she try using the three questions above to note events and thoughts about what was happening and what she was learning. She suggested Samina 'mind mapped' it on a side of A4 paper to show her learning (see Figure 2.3).

There may be times when you have felt that you have done a lot but not been sure what you have learnt. Maybe you have even resented the fact you have been 'used as a pair of hands' to get the work done or felt that the environment was not conducive for learning. In response to a recommendation in the Francis Report (2013), The National Institute for Health and Care Excellence (NICE) has issued a guideline advising organisations of safe staffing levels, which is intended to ensure that the right number of nurses with the right skills are in the right place at the right time (National Quality Board, 2013). This guideline is approximate and describes a minimum number of nurses, which would vary according to the degree of dependence of the patients cared for. For example, in high-dependency units, the ratio of nurses to patients will be no more than two patients to each nurse, whereas in an acute adult ward the minimum number is no more than eight patients to each nurse. Factors such as supervising students and mentorship responsibilities are acknowledged as fundamental aspects of a nurses' role and may result in a requirement for additional numbers of nurses to maintain safe staffing levels. One key recommendation identified in the Francis Report (2013) is that each patient will have a named nurse and ward managers will work in a supervisory capacity. If you ever feel that these standards are not being met, it is important that you raise your concerns. There are ways, however, to 'see' what you are learning

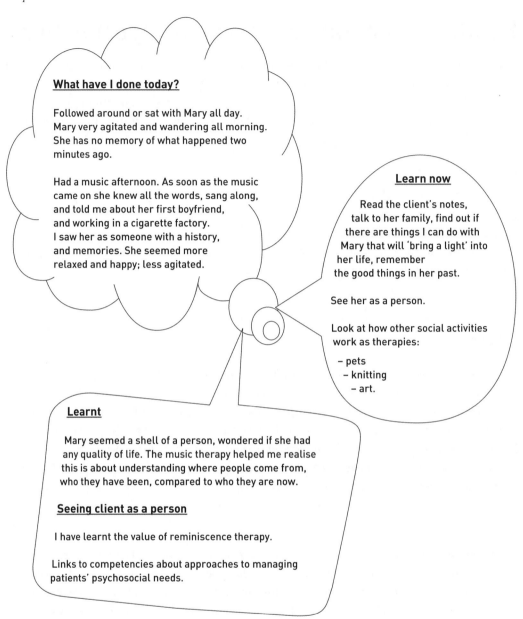

Figure 2.3: Mind-mapping reflection

about nursing people from nearly all of your practice experiences and how you are adapting common practices to different individual needs. You might try the following ways to learn:

- teach another student or carer;

- give handover and answer queries about your patient;

- work alongside another student from a different discipline and share your ideas about the patient's care; how your roles complement and differ from each other's;

- escort patients to investigations and procedures;

- shadow other healthcare professionals;
- visit agencies who provide specialist support;
- spend a day with a porter and get their perspective;
- undertake a peer review with another student.

Make the most of your supernumerary status while you are a student and activate your learning. Prior to and at the end of each period of learning ask yourself the following questions.

- What were my aims and objectives?
- How well did I achieve my objectives?
- What do I still need to do?
- Were there any factors I hadn't considered that influenced my learning:
  - o that I could have done something about – prevention or action?
  - o that were unavoidable?

Summarise your experiences and record them in your portfolio. There are different versions of personal development plan templates available. However, most plans will have a set of components which culminate in your short- and long-term goals for clinical and non-clinical learning.

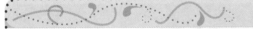

Chapter summary

This chapter has overviewed how a PDP might be useful in directing your learning. We hope that you will take away four key points:

- a SWOT analysis will help you identify your learning needs;
- using the learning styles questionnaire might help you identify which teaching and learning methods you are most comfortable with;
- using the steps in completing a personal development plan will enable you to plan and focus activities for a piece of learning to overcome any gaps or weaknesses you have identified;
- you need to capture your learning from your everyday practice experience, analyse what you are learning from it and what you still have to learn.

As in Chapter 1, we have referred to several ways you can use to show your learning and the evidence you might collect. Chapter 3 will address some of these in more depth.

Further reading

Francis, R (2013) *Report of the Mid Staffordshire NHS Foundation Trust Public Inquiry: Executive summary.* London: Stationery Office.

A detailed review into patient safety and the quality of patient care within the NHS.

Frankel, A (2009) Nurses' learning styles: promoting better integration of theory into practice. *Nursing Times*, 105 (2): 24–7.

An accessible review of the topic.

Honey, P and Mumford, DA (2000) *The Learning Styles Helper's Guide.* Maidenhead: Peter Honey Publications.

Defines and describes which self-assessment questionnaire is best for you to identify your learning style.

Hutchfield, K (2010) *Information for Nursing Students.* Exeter: Learning Matters.

A practical and clear guide to mastering information skills; explains how to plan and implement a search for information and make judgements on the quality of sources found.

National Quality Board/ NHS England (2013) *How to Ensure the Right People, with the Right Skills, are in the Right Place at the Right Time: A guide to nursing and midwifery and care staffing capacity and capability.* Available at: www.england.nhs.uk/wp-content/uploads/2013/11/nqb-how-to-guid.pdf

A guide to nursing and midwifery staffing capacity and capability.

NICE (2013) *Safe Staffing for Nursing in Acute Hospitals.* London: National Institute for Health and Care Excellence.

University of Salford Faculty of Health and Social Care (2007) *Personal Development Planning Resources Pack.*

Provides a comprehensive but easy-to-use guide for personal development planning with explanations about five steps to produce a plan shown clearly on p8 of the pack.

Useful websites

www.palgrave.com/studentstudyskills/page/Useful-resources/
This site has details of Stella Cottrell's *Skills for Success* (2015) and many other resources for personal development planning.

www.peterhoney.com
Peter Honey's website for learning styles.

Chapter 3
Collecting evidence for your portfolio

Chapter aims

After reading this chapter you will be able to:

- identify the skills that are necessary for building an effective portfolio;
- identify the sort of evidence to keep in your portfolio, and select the best to show your progress;
- understand what is meant by critical thinking;
- start keeping a reflective diary for your portfolio.

Introduction

In the last chapter we focused on how to assess your learning needs and produce a personal development plan. This chapter provides you with a skills starter kit for putting together a portfolio, and explores what sort of evidence to keep in your portfolio. The chapter then introduces the idea of keeping a reflective diary, and shows how you can also begin to use this to help your learning and development right from the start of your programme. You will have seen from Chapter 2 and the section on learning styles that we all learn in different ways; this may indicate that we lean towards using particular kinds of evidence and avoid others. You need to be able to use a broad range of evidence for different purposes, including descriptive evidence, critical analysis and discussion of practice, self-assessment and evidence of feedback from others.

The key skills necessary for building an effective portfolio are:

- discriminating what actually is valid evidence for inserting in your portfolio;
- finding out where to locate such evidence;
- identifying the key people to help you capture the evidence;
- keeping a reflective diary.

Skills needed for putting your portfolio together

This chapter introduces you to Rachel, who has just completed the first year of her Pre-registration Nursing Programme in the adult field of practice. Rachel shares her experiences and the challenges she encountered in developing a variety of skills to put her portfolio together. The skills Rachel describes are examples that are necessary to compile an effective portfolio. The level, ability and competence of skills are individual and variable so students are often stronger in some and weaker in others. The important point is to build on those skills you identify as weak.

Case study: Rachel's skills starter kit for putting together a successful portfolio

Here is a list of some of the key skills I found necessary for compiling and maintaining a successful portfolio:

- the ability to write clear, succinct, comprehensive summaries;
- IT skills;
- distinguishing between direct and indirect evidence;
- an ability to describe, analyse (and reflect on) my patient care experiences.

In order to develop my portfolio over my first year I had to think about why each of the above was important. I found it helpful to share this with the other students in my tutorial group. You might want to add your own thoughts to mine as you read my explanations below.

The ability to write clear, succinct, comprehensive summaries to introduce each piece or package of evidence in my portfolio

This was invaluable in clarifying, with my personal tutor and my mentor, how well I achieved each of my NMC competencies. This helped me to use time in meetings with my mentor and personal tutor constructively. I was able to find materials quickly in order to sum up my learning and plan for my second year. In order to make my portfolio manageable my aim was to identify material through clear explanation of each section. I started by updating everything I had already collected, sorting it out so that it reflected what I felt were important patient care experiences whilst I was on practice, and what I had learnt from them. (I also made sure I made copies of the materials in case anything got lost.)

Using basic IT skills to house materials and to create electronic files in my portfolio

This made my portfolio more accessible for everyone. I also felt it was quite a sophisticated format and great for remote use when I am away from the university campus. At times when I was expected to learn on my own I found being aware of search engines and knowing how to using a computer proved useful for independent study and finding information. Although I wouldn't say I was highly skilled in IT, recent telecommunications technology enabled me to use a range of interactive learning tools to create and support the content of my evidence.

(E-portfolios are discussed in more detail in Chapter 4.)

continued ...

continued ...

Distinguishing between direct and indirect evidence

This was important for putting materials into different categories and sections in my portfolio. I first had to be sure that I understood the difference between indirect and direct evidence. My personal tutor helped me define each type as follows.

- Indirect evidence includes extracts, excerpts and transcripts from my reflective diaries and personal reflective practice exercises with my mentor. I found mind mapping a really useful tool for summarising my reflective discussions with my mentor and other students.
- Direct evidence can be identified as that which reflects direct observation of my practice performance, such as statements provided by expert practitioners and service users. For example, the activities during my placement experience and clinical assessments by my mentor provided me with comments and guidance from clinical staff about how I am doing and where I can improve or further develop my skills.

Critical analysis of and reflection on my practice

This was harder to learn. It took me a while to understand that I couldn't just describe the patient care experiences I had participated in with my mentor and others. I had to learn to ask questions about the patient care I was giving rather than just accept and copy what my mentors did as 'the best way to do things'. My mentor and personal tutor gave me some good tips on different tools I could use for this and the university had a reusable learning object on reflection and a virtual portfolio tool that were really helpful in getting me started.

(See Useful websites section at the end of this chapter.)

Activity 3.1   *Reflection*

Review the list of skills above that were identified by Rachel as necessary to complete her portfolio. Which of the skills are you most confident about? Make a note of any future skills you need to focus on to compare developing an e-portfolio with a paper-based portfolio.

Critical thinking and portfolio writing

One of the key skills to be developed in pre-registration nursing students has been identified by the NMC as *Critical analysis and critical thinking*.

The word 'critical' in this context is not negative (as in the sense of being critical of someone) but is more about examining and questioning some types of information and evidence. Price and Harrington (2013) propose several different meanings of critical thinking:

In the clinical context, critical carries connotation of risk and the need for urgent intervention. In the academic context, critical takes on several different meanings and it is apparent that to be critical can be different things dependent on the teaching or assessment involved. (p2)

A competent nurse will make many judgements and decisions throughout the day, and Price and Harrington (2013) link critical thinking in their definition as follows:

A competent nurse is one who develops powers of analysis and investigation; is able to select relevant information, to plan a course of action and then judge what is best to do in a given circumstance. The nurse has to be competent to manage risk. (p2)

Learning activities you undertake to develop your evidence

Throughout your portfolio you will be required to demonstrate that you have closely examined information and approaches to care which underpin the patient care skills you learn in your placements. Critical thinking is about examining whether or not there is adequate evidence for accepting that knowledge or a clinical skill is correct. Most people rarely question or challenge routine procedures, often relying on other people to think for them instead of thinking for themselves. However, developing critical thinking is about you learning how to question routine skills and possibly eliminating certain tasks, even coming up with creative, new and useful suggestions. This means accepting, rejecting or suspending judgement about a routine skill until you have considered all aspects and information available. Critical thinking requires you to keep an open mind and to arrive at logical decisions which are based on the best available evidence. Fisher and Scriven (1997) define critical thinking as *skilled, active, interpretation and evaluation of observations, communication and information and argumentation* (p21).

In critical thinking, you consider the available evidence about a skill or piece of knowledge and evaluate its strength. However, if step-by-step examination of the skill or piece of knowledge results in no definite decision, then the judgement may be suspended as inconclusive. Irrespective of the knowledge or skill being examined, a critical thinker would:

- raise questions about whether things are appropriate and safe, or whether they could be improved;
- assess evidence available on the internet or in journals, or observe expert practice where there is no (as yet) published material;
- interpret information set out in the evidence;

- test conclusions against standards and relevant criteria;
- be aware of intuitive (gut feeling) responses such as perceptions about things.

A critical thinker would then consider the skill or piece of knowledge with an open mind before accepting, rejecting or suspending judgements and conclusions.

Activity 3.2   *Critical thinking*

Identify a skill or routine procedure which has been the norm during a placement experience. Consider the points listed above for critical thinking. Gather information about the skill from the internet, clinical guidelines and from journals, etc. Is the method of completing the skill or procedure appropriate, inappropriate or inconclusive?

Case study: Questioning routine decisions and making judgements

Rachel selected the following exercise to help her to understand the rationale behind some of the judgements and decisions around administering drugs to chronically ill patients. After examining the evidence on the internet, Rachel referred to the points in the list above and determined that self-administration for some chronically ill patients is something that could be improved. Rachel found the recent government reports which encourage self-medication for people with chronic conditions helpful, as well as several articles on how to assess patient readiness and ability to self-administer. Rachel led a group seminar to discuss the merits of patient self-administration.

Activity 3.3   *Communication*

Begin with your own action set or working group comprising student representatives from each field of nursing including adult, mental health, learning disabilities and children's nursing. Using articles and information collected from the internet, lead a group discussion/ seminar on the merits of patient self-administration of medication.

Rachel discussed the issue with her mentor, who agreed to complete a risk assessment on some patients to identify whether they are suitable for teaching self-administration. After a trial run, including patient teaching and safety procedures, the change was made and some patients who routinely had nurses to administer their drugs were able to be self-medicating. This made them happy and more independent. Rachel also developed evidence for her portfolio.

The sort of evidence you should include in your portfolio

Examples of the sort of evidence to keep in your portfolio are records and materials which demonstrate that you are competent in performing tasks and safe patient care.

As portfolios are increasingly used as part of assessment, it is crucial that the evidence you collect is valid. An external examiner may request to review your portfolio to confirm your learning achievements, and part of the process will be to review the validity of the evidence provided.

Where you might find valid evidence

The sources of evidence it is appropriate to use for your portfolio may not at first be directly obvious. It can be a little tricky to identify what is real, valid evidence and what constitutes materials of interest.

Rachel describes below some examples of evidence she inserted in her portfolio.

- Case studies: In my portfolio I used a case study to demonstrate my competence in direct patient care. The case study, put simply, is a care plan that is written in essay form. The essay included a comprehensive account of social, physical and psychological care with vital information about a patient and their family. I was also able to show my involvement in work activities with a multidisciplinary team. Here is an outline of the patient case study I inserted in my portfolio.

Example of a patient case study

Robert is a 59-year-old draughtsman who has been admitted with a cough, wheezing and difficulty with breathing. Robert has been a heavy smoker for a number of years and also consumes alcohol regularly with his friends. An examination of his chest and a series of investigations including a chest X-ray, sputum test and blood gases were ordered by the physician. A diagnosis of asthma and exacerbation of chronic bronchitis was made. The full case study included a patient nursing assessment, nursing interventions, physiotherapy, evaluation of care and medical treatments.

Collectively, the case study above demonstrated Rachel's competence and involvement in nursing activities and skills to keep as records in her portfolio.

It is outside the remit of this book to provide all details of the full case study, but you can review a variety of other case study examples by using the links given at the end of this chapter.

- Application of the 6Cs to nursing care: Referring back to the table in Chapter 1, I selected a variety and range of behaviours which were relevant to include in the case study example about Robert.

- Due to Robert's diagnosis of asthma and bronchitis I identified that it was important to be aware of evidence-based practice for caring for a patient with respiratory problems. I noted that there were also specific skills which would be necessary for effectively communicating with a breathless patient, in particular, being approachable, developing a rapport and careful listening would be helpful. As Robert had a history of alcohol abuse and heavy smoking I made a note of the need for compassion to treat him with dignity, humanity, respect and kindness. Although not obviously relevant at first sight, courage in demonstrating integrity and ethical practice, commitment to providing a safe and positive culture, and being open and responsive with displaying honesty and candour would become apparent in dealing with Robert and his family.

- Integrated care pathways: I included an integrated care pathway in my portfolio as an example of my practice learning activities. An integrated care pathway or ICP, as it has become known, is a multidisciplinary outline of care placed in an appropriate timeframe. The ICP shows a patient journey from assessment through to discharge and all the care delivered in between. The ICP is evidence-based to ensure that up-to-date care is delivered. The achievement of outcomes is measured to evaluate how effective the care has been. In the event that a piece of care is not delivered as expected, this is termed a variance. An example of a variance might be when a patient is not discharged from hospital on the date planned because of a urinary infection following catheterisation post-operatively. Including the patient care pathway in my portfolio with reflection and discussion about my performance provided evidence of my experience in assessment and care planning, and showed some involvement in patient daily-living activities.

It is outside the remit of this book to provide templates and examples of care pathways. There are many examples of ICPs available in the literature, and links to some are provided at the end of this chapter.

- Reflective account/patient story: A reflective account or patient story is a record of a piece of care or an extract from a learning experience in my student journey. The record I inserted in my portfolio indicated my thoughts at the time and my identified strengths, weaknesses and limitations. The account provides insight into my structured and unstructured learning experiences.

- Audit reports: Audits are completed to provide information about care delivery in accordance with set standards. Criteria are measured to show compliance with standards and guidelines, and any gaps and omissions are noted. This information can then be used to focus any developments or resources to make necessary improvements. I used the extracts from clinical audit reports recorded in my portfolio to show my involvement and experience in clinical quality and improving standards of patient care.

Clinical skills

Be very clear about your NMC competencies for each placement. Familiarise yourself with your clinical assessment document (CAD) and criteria for assessment of skills. Your ongoing achievement record (OAR)/clinical assessment document will provide a record for your mentor to judge your professional competence. It will be reviewed by academic staff and an external examiner in an examination board meeting to confirm your progress. Meet with your mentor to discuss your learning needs. Throughout your placement experience there will be progress meetings with your mentor and link teacher. Use each meeting to explore the learning opportunities and match them to your learning outcomes. Find out what materials can be used as evidence of practice learning activities.

Simulated clinical experience

The NMC recognises simulated learning as part of the curriculum practice hours. Simulation came into being to help in the shortage of placement experiences available for students. As a teaching and learning strategy, simulation is effective and is often combined with virtual learning and technology. Virtual learning communities are used in some programmes to guide multi-disciplinary teams to achieve learning outcomes together, especially where capacity for placements is limited. Students are often provided with a selection of problem-based scenarios which can be used to demonstrate competence in a range and variety of different clinical situations. The experience can then be verified by a lecturer. Rachel inserted each record of simulated experience into her portfolio. One example is evidence of her learning achievements in cardiopulmonary resuscitation techniques.

Mandatory training

Mandatory training is compulsory and a legal requirement. The requirement includes lifting and moving, resuscitation, fire training and infection control. Each person is presented with a certificate of attendance to confirm that they have received the training. An annual update is also a legal requirement. Rachel filed each certificate of attendance in her portfolio as evidence of the learning activities in mandatory training.

Clinical governance/clinical risk reports

Clinical governance assessments and reports are written by clinical staff. The key elements of clinical governance include risk management, leadership and quality. Each element is assessed and the process for achieving standards reviewed against policies and guidelines. Any reports of deficits, including financial or training, can comprise evidence of your involvement in clinical governance. Should an accident or incident occur, a risk assessment and report are generated. These reports provide a good source of evidence and Rachel has filed them in relevant sections of her portfolio.

The list of evidence sources above are examples only and many more could be identified just as there will be many people who can help you to locate and capture the evidence. Such people include your mentor, personal teacher, link lecturer, clinical manager, academic staff and members of the multidisciplinary team. Their involvement may not always be apparent and overt but be aware that most times they will be pleased to advise you and direct you to materials.

Activity 3.4   *Reflection*

Review your list of learning achievements. What other evidence can you think of? What, where and who might help you to capture valid evidence?

Reflection and portfolio writing

The activities of questioning values and beliefs, referred to as critical thinking in the previous section, are also involved in reflection. Reflection is another key skill that is developed by, and essential to, the successful portfolio. One of the benefits of a portfolio noted at the beginning of this book is that it provides a record of knowledge that is identified from reflecting on practice. Reflection and **reflective practice** are now part of teaching and learning strategies for all nursing programmes, and you will hear the terms on a number of occasions in the classroom and in your placements for a variety of situations throughout your student journey. We often take experiences in our stride as part of our everyday lives with few of us considering whether there might be other possibilities and different responses we might have applied to improve a situation. The process of reflection helps us to do this. Howatson-Jones (2013, p6) defines reflection as: *A way of examining your experience in order to look for the possibility of other explanations and alternative ways of doing things.* She adds: *What is required is an open and enquiring mind that can accept the possibility of different explanations.*

Reflection is not seen as unusual. Howatson-Jones believes that we all do this whenever we have mental or physical space to take a moment to think about things. Reflection, she states, *can help to affirm as well as correct actions,* adding: *There are benefits of reflection for individual effectiveness, improving problem-solving skills of the workforce and for enhancing patient care* (Howatson-Jones, 2013, p6).

An example of considering other possibly better ways of doing things can be illustrated by this example of planning a journey.

> ### Scenario: Reflection-on-action
>
> *You decide to take a flight from Glasgow to Birmingham on the basis that you always took that route before and you arrived at the destination a little delayed but safe and sound, and at a reasonable cost. Consider taking time to reflect on your experience: would the time and cost of the journey be comparable, or could you even improve on your travel time (as well as on the cost), if you went by car or train?*

This activity is called **reflection-on-action** and involves a type of reflection often seen as early as the first and second year of the pre-registration programme. Better ways of doing things may not always be highly visible and obvious to us, so we opt instead for the known, existing and safer ways. Schön (1984) also identifies another type of reflection, **reflection-in-action**, which involves reflecting on the action at the same time as you are doing it. This is a more advanced skill that you are more likely to do when you have more experience, perhaps during your final placement experience.

Kolb's experiential cycle and reflection

According to Kolb (1984), reflection is an essential element of learning. This is illustrated in what he refers to as an experiential learning cycle. The cycle follows a clockwise direction, as shown in Figure 3.1, and demonstrates continuing attempts to find ways of improving.

Activity 3.5   *Reflection*

Identify an experience or event, for example a task or care activity from your first practice module, and apply the reflection-on-action process. Think about what you did and how you did it, and what your thoughts and feelings were at the time. Consider new ideas and different alternative approaches with your mentor. How could the skill or task have been improved?

If you can, experiment with a new idea in a safe environment and under supervision of your mentor. Try out your new idea as a result of earlier learning.

This process of updating and reviewing your learning in Activity 3.5 forces you to step back and see the bigger picture, and will be a defining moment in your study activities. Reflection shows us how we can do things better next time, often simply by looking with a fresh pair of eyes at a situation. Therefore, reflection should be an activity recorded in your portfolio as a way of helping develop your learning and understanding how to improve your practice. In today's rapidly changing healthcare settings, the reflective part of your portfolio will help to demonstrate that you do not take routine at face value, but are aware of the need to review and constantly improve your work. With the focus on cost savings, your portfolio will help you demonstrate your awareness of the importance of planning and resources needed to reach your goals.

One way of recording your reflections and reviews of events in your portfolio is to use a personal reflective diary or log. This will be considered in more detail later in the chapter.

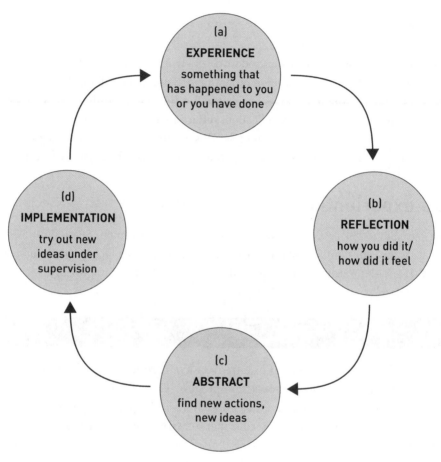

Figure 3.1: Kolb's cycle of experiential learning
(Source: Kolb, 1984)

How keeping a reflective diary fits with your portfolio

A reflective diary or journal is a popular learning tool to record daily events and incidents and to explore what you thought about them or how they affected you. The diary provides a means of discussing your fears and anxieties, and the format for sharing experiences with your colleagues in a non-threatening way. The diary is personal to you and need not be shown to anyone if you prefer it that way; however, as part of your learning activities it will comprise an important part of your portfolio. Write only what you want, when you want. Describe key events in your practice placement. Your diary should be written honestly as it will provide a useful record of your thoughts, feelings and opinions, so report both positive and negative things. There are no set ways to reflect or record your diary and you will gradually build your own approach to doing things in a way that suits you. You may find it helpful to list a set of questions to focus your thinking, similar to those shown in the box below.

Get into the habit of collecting records and information for your diary. Use the list of questions in the box below to focus your thoughts to enter in your diary on a regular basis.

Developing a reflective diary

The following list of questions may help you to focus your thoughts as a starting point in developing your reflective diary to keep in your portfolio.

- What happened/what did you do? What went well? What went not so well?
- Do you feel comfortable about what happened? Reflect on the whole experience.
- What did you learn? Can you make sense of it?
- How successful were you? What are you aiming for?
- How can you bring the learning into your daily work activities/your NMC learning outcomes and competencies?
- What are your next steps? Has it changed the way you will do things in the future?

Activity 3.6 — *Reflection*

Consider an event or incident from your last placement experience. Review the questions listed above and commence writing your reflective diary. Insert your diary in your portfolio.

Your university may provide you with a template to use for your journal. If not, then you can use the list of questions above. Use a fresh list each time and record a new sheet to keep in your portfolio. It's your own private record – enjoy it.

Organising and presenting your portfolio

How you organise your portfolio may be predetermined by your university. Alternatively, you may be free to design your own structure. A logical flow would be:

- an introduction, to you and what you want to learn/need to learn;

- key documents verifying your learning (assessment documents);

- evidence supporting learning;

- other relevant material (see Table 3.1).

One way to organise your evidence could be according to the NMC domains (see Concept summary below). Another would be in relation to the aims and objectives in your personal development plan (see Case study that follows).

Concept summary: Four domains for competence (NMC, 2010c)

1. Professional values.
2. Communication and interpersonal skills.
3. Nursing practice and decision making.
4. Leadership, management and team working.

Case study

Remember Natasha (from Chapter 1)? She is a mature student with elderly parents, one of whom requires 24-hour care at home. As an adult nursing student her first practice experience was in a busy male orthopaedic ward. She was looking forward to getting to grips with fundamental care skills, hoping to pass one of the essential care skills assessments and learn how to plan care for people with orthopaedic problems. Her concerns were about how she would feel nursing older men, particularly if the disability was long term. After speaking to her mentor she realised that many of the men had long-standing orthopaedic conditions. Natasha was experiencing some difficulty in divorcing herself from her worries about her father. By the end of her placement experience Natasha had been able to add two unexpected aspects of learning to her portfolio – one about the patients' needs regarding 'living with disability' and the other about managing her own emotional needs relating to the situation with her father (professional values). This is reflected in the final column of Table 3.1.

Natasha realised that her learning needed to broaden out to encompass a more holistic perspective about the patient experience. In doing so she found that she did need to try out making a reflective note on two aspects of her practice experience, as well as keeping records of her clinical activities.

continued ...

continued ...

... continued

Introduction	• Purpose of the portfolio • Stage of course • Course requirements for this stage • Placements • Personal development or action plan • Learning summary for period and how that relates to evidence in portfolio	**Natasha's end of semester one portfolio** *Just finished my first placement and first semester. Working on an acute male orthopaedic ward. Aim was to get my fundamental care skills up to scratch and get at least one of my ESCs out of the way. Didn't realise how much caring for men on this ward would challenge me emotionally. Learnt a lot about becoming 'disabled' and people having to adjust to disability, and the team involved in their care.*
Key assessment documents to insert in your portfolio • Ongoing achievement record • Assessment of practice record • (Moves from one placement experience to another to show my mentors how I am progressing.)		**Achieved level** = two on the scale for most competencies **Outstanding** ones still to complete: vulnerable people legislation 1.3/2.6 health promotion 3.1.1/3.3.1/4.2 care planning

continued ...

Evidence of learning	**Sections** From action plan aims; by NMC domain; by type of evidence	**Development of clinical skills – section one** Diary notes 1–5, witness statements 1, 2 ESC 1 achieved; training on hoists **Understanding disability – section two** Reflection 1 **Understanding personal/professional boundaries – section three** Reflective diary with mentor
Records of theoretical progress OSCE Personal academic record		**Theory – section four** Assignment feedback – passed sociology/psychology essay Passed clinical exam on hand washing (OSCE 1) and basic observations (OSCE 2)
Action plan for next semester/ placement	Move to the front of your portfolio for each semester so that the most recent learning is at the front Include curriculum vitae and any other relevant materials	Feel confident at meeting activities of daily living but I need more experience in: 1. communication – including aids for hearing / speech deficits; 2. medicines management – including calculation and administration; 3. have seen an admission procedure but not done one on my own; 4. not yet had chance to write a patient care pathway; 5. need more practice in handover reports; 6. must use theory to underpin my practice.

Table 3.1: Structuring your portfolio

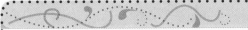

Chapter summary

First, this chapter has introduced you to the skills you will need to compile a successful portfolio. Some of these skills, such as critical analysis and reflection, are skills you will need in your everyday work as a nurse. Second, the chapter has looked at what types of evidence are appropriate to keep in your portfolio. Some of these may not at first appear to be directly obvious. There are also materials which may be of interest, but which will not be important to demonstrate your competence for assessment purposes. Finally, we have looked at the reflective diary, a useful tool to keep in your portfolio. You can use this for recording personal and professional experiences and feelings. Eventually, you will be able to look back and see how you have grown in your journey as a student nurse.

Having worked through this chapter, you should now be aware that it is important to identify which skills you already feel you are competent in and note those which require further development. You will also be aware that not all materials comprise valid evidence to keep in your portfolio. The next chapter will reintroduce you to the idea of compiling an e-portfolio.

Further reading

Fisher, A and Scriven, M (1997) *Critical Thinking: Its definition and assessment.* Norwich: University of East Anglia, Centre for Research in Critical Thinking.

Defines critical thinking and provides an account of the competencies involved.

Howatson-Jones, L (2013) *Reflective Practice in Nursing* (2nd edition). London: SAGE Publications.

Provides succinct definition of reflection and describes the process.

Kolb, DA (1984) *Experiential Learning: Experience as the source of learning and development.* Upper Saddle River, NJ.

Kolb created his famous experiential model out of four elements of concrete experience, observation and reflection, forming abstract concepts and testing them in new situations.

Price, B and Harrington, A (2013) *Critical Thinking and Writing for Nursing Students* (2nd edition). London: SAGE Publications.

Provides an accessible introduction to a subject that can be daunting. See especially Chapter 2, Reflecting, and Chapter 10, Building and using your portfolio of learning.

Schön, D (1984) *The Reflective Practitioner: How professionals think in action.* London: Temple Smith.

This book shows how professionals really go about solving problems. Schön maintains that to meet the challenges of their work, professionals rely on learning from practice rather than in the classroom. He describes reflection-on-action as analysing their reaction to an experience, and exploring reasons and consequences of their actions. Reflection-in-action, for more advanced professionals, is described as learning which occurs during or at the same time as the action takes place.

Useful websites

http://pathways.nice.org.uk
Page from NICE, giving access to different pathways and guidance.

www.icptoolkit.org/home.aspx
A mental health integrated care pathways toolkit produced by NHS Scotland.

Chapter 4
Using your portfolio to demonstrate achievement

> ## NMC Standards for Pre-registration Nursing Education
>
> This chapter will address the following competencies:
>
> **Domain 1: Professional values**
>
> 7. All nurses must be responsible and accountable for keeping their knowledge and skills up to date through continuing professional development. They must aim to improve their performance and enhance the safety and quality of care through evaluation, supervision and appraisal.
> 8. All nurses must practise independently, recognising the limits of their competence and knowledge. They must reflect on these limits and seek advice from, or refer to, other professionals where necessary.
>
> **Domain 2: Communication and interpersonal skills**
>
> 7. All nurses must maintain accurate, clear and complete records, including the use of electronic formats, using appropriate and plain language.
> 8. All nurses must respect individual rights to confidentiality and keep information secure and confidential in accordance with the law and relevant ethical and regulatory frameworks, taking account of local protocols. They must also actively share personal information with others when the interests of safety and protection override the need for confidentiality.

> ## Chapter aims
>
> After reading this chapter you will be able to:
>
> - describe how your portfolio can be used to demonstrate your achievement of NMC standards and competencies;
> - identify valid work samples to demonstrate competence;
> - explain how the essential skills clusters can help you to map your growth in competence;
>
> *continued ...*

continued ....

- understand how you can use your portfolio to showcase evidence of learning activities in preparation for progression meetings with your mentor;
- appreciate the e-portfolio as an effective vehicle for keeping evidence of your learning;
- link your portfolio to NMC essential skills and competency domains learning.

Introduction

This chapter is about using your portfolio to demonstrate your competence. In it, you will be introduced to Robbie, a mature student who is in the second year of a pre-registration mental health programme. Robbie shares his student journey, in particular how he used his portfolio to demonstrate competence and how he found NMC standards, competencies and essential skills useful in focusing his competency achievements. Robbie has opted to use the e-portfolio as a means of housing his evidence and he provides some helpful tips on making this successful.

During your programme you will be expected to meet your mentor and personal tutor regularly, and possibly an external examiner may request a meeting. It is crucial that your portfolio show-cases your competence achievements in an organised and structured way in preparation for these progression meetings.

Using your portfolio to demonstrate achievement of the NMC competencies

Definitions of competence include a range of skills which are recognised in the NMC domains – see Chapter 3. Your assessment of practice document and grading criteria will probably be based on your university levels of competency scheme.

Activity 4.1 *Critical thinking*

Ask members of your family and make a note of what you yourself believe a nurse does and what a nurse is. Look at various definitions on the internet and compare what you can identify as key differences.

You can find some definitions on the following websites:

- www.nmc-uk.org;
- www.rcn.org.uk;
- www.icn.ch/who-we-are/icn-definition-of-nursing/.

Behind a smooth, competent performance in any task relating to patient care, there are aspects of knowledge, skills and attitudes relating to the activity. Achieving a competent and smooth performance requires some or each of the following.

- Skills acquisition: this requires approved clinical placements when your mentors will spend time organising learning activities to achieve your competencies. Alternatively, some competencies may be achieved in simulated learning sessions that are arranged by your academic staff.

- Skills development: this requires you to observe your mentor demonstrating a skill, then opportunities for you to practise the skill under the supervision of your mentor until you feel confident.

- Assessment of your performance: this requires a mentor in each clinical area who has undergone specific training to provide a supervisory role and also to complete your practice assessments. Other (non-nursing) staff may also contribute to your practice learning and assessment once they have been suitably prepared. However, during the last 12 weeks of your programme, only a sign-off mentor is allowed to confirm your competence.

The sign-off mentor is someone:

- whose name appears on a local mentor register;
- who has completed an annual update;
- who has completed a triennial review if on the mentor register for three years;
- who is from a similar care background as yourself.

In some aspects of your programme you may be required to assess yourself. Once your competency assessment has been completed, recorded and signed by your mentor, you should insert it in the relevant section of your portfolio. As discussed in Chapter 2, it will help you to prepare for your progression meetings with your mentor if you have written summaries of each piece of evidence.

As an example of a summary for a piece of evidence, let's look at patient teaching. Your summary would include the following.

- From your collection of research articles underpinning patient teaching you would need a paragraph on effective teaching and learning in the clinical setting.

- Then you would add a short précis about skills you performed under the supervision of your mentor. These might include creating an effective environment or demonstration of the procedure to the patient, giving the patient an opportunity to ask any questions or raise any concerns.

- Notes about the interpersonal aspect of the session.

- Assessment of your competence and any comments made by your mentor about your performance.

- Your own reflection of the teaching session – what went well and what could have gone better and why.

Activity 4.2 | *Reflection*

Identify any skill you performed when caring for a patient who is being discharged from hospital to their own home in the community. An example might be teaching the patient one (or several) daily living activities. Make a note of the various skills and tasks involved. The summary can be added to your portfolio.

Although the answers to this activity will be personal to you, Robbie has shared some of the key points of his answers below. You may find this helpful in structuring your own thoughts.

Case study: Robbie's example of some of the key points of Activity 4.2

The activity I have selected for this example is teaching Ed, an elderly gentleman who is soon to be discharged home, how to complete his personal hygiene when he is at home. Ed has depression and is partially sighted.

- I selected a quiet area in the ward as a suitable environment for the teaching to take place.
- I put Ed at ease and gave him a full explanation of personal hygiene skills.
- I asked Ed what aspects of personal hygiene he can already manage and feels confident about completing and what he needs help with.
- I identified the components of teaching, including searching for knowledge and relevant articles to underpin personal hygiene on the internet.
- I demonstrated personal hygiene skills to Ed.
- I checked out Ed's understanding of what he must do.
- I provided an opportunity for Ed to demonstrate personal hygiene under my supervision.
- I gave Ed constructive feedback on the effectiveness of his performance.
- Ed did at times still appear anxious and agitated about what to do. He did have difficulty remembering, so I applied important strategies such as reassurance and clarification of his uncertainties and repeated the demonstration. Eventually, Ed was able to complete his personal hygiene unaided in preparation for his discharge home.
- I made a note of how I felt the teaching activity went and identified several areas I can improve on.

Creating valid and reliable examples of evidence for your portfolio

The introduction of portfolio assessment is one strategy which has helped to provide the assessment of broader and wider-ranging activities and clinical experiences. An example of this is the patient journey. It is important that all of the contents in your portfolio are kept confidential, so always keep in mind who it is for, who will be looking at it and who will have access to it. Any patient or family details in documents must be anonymised. It is also important that you feel ownership of it. It is your work, and you decide what goes where and when.

Some examples of evidence that you might include in your portfolio to demonstrate achievement of your competencies are given below.

Evidence from academic work to increase your understanding of patient care

Assignments or patient care studies which explain the physical, psychological and social aspects of the patient and family

This is academic work you might include in your portfolio to demonstrate competence in completing a nursing assessment, care requirements and evaluation of outcomes of care delivered.

Grades from formal examinations which focus on a practice-based approach

For example, objective structured clinical examinations (OSCEs) representing various scenarios using real patients can be used to verify your competence in problem solving and decision making.

Evidence from reflective exercises to help you to review experience and consider better ways of doing things

Descriptions of your participation and understanding of evidence-based patient care pathways, demonstrating a patient journey set in a time frame with multidisciplinary evidence-based care and identified variances when care did not go according to expectations

An account of how you participated in such a patient journey, and your reflection on it, can be included in your portfolio to demonstrate competence in evidence-based practice, multidisciplinary working, patient assessment and evaluation of care outcomes. As referred to earlier in this chapter, all patient care documents must be anonymised, with any details of individual patients removed.

Reflective pieces, which through experience of reflecting in or on actions may indicate a better or more improved approach to patient care

Using critical thinking and reflective practice skills, including mind maps, annotated care plans and other work which involves finding evidence or facts, may provide a better way of working.

Evidence from project work done to increase your knowledge and understanding of team work and problem solving

This can include selected practice-based learning scenarios to show your team-working skills and collaborative working activities. It may also be used to demonstrate managing teams, teaching patients and team members, and delegation of tasks to other people. Experience of team meetings, patient handover reports and multidisciplinary team-care study discussions can confirm your involvement in working with other healthcare professionals (see Rachel's project in Chapter 3).

Evidence from quality assurance activities

Reports and results of audits of patient care can be used to demonstrate your participation in quality assurance activities and care improvement strategies.

Evidence from direct observation and the assessment of NMC competencies

Assessment of NMC competencies by your mentor within your clinical placements can be used to demonstrate competence in the combination of knowledge, performance, skills and attitudes.

The above list provides only a few examples of some of the work samples you might use to demonstrate your assessed competence. By combining all of the methods above into patient care plans or patient care pathways and inserting them into your portfolio, you will be able to capture learning over time in a way that other types of tests may not. Your portfolio is an effective and acceptable way to demonstrate your competence and show how you have applied new skills and knowledge in your placements to your mentors, personal teachers and external examiners.

Alternative formats for your portfolio

Each university has its own ideas about portfolio structure and sequence of content to provide you with guidance for organising material. Having said that, you will find there is an NMC requirement for specific learning outcomes to be met at each stage of your programme. This requirement will undoubtedly result in similarity between students as to types of evidence you select and your decisions of what goes into your portfolio, but do not be concerned if your work does not strictly follow the same pattern as someone else's. Aimee, Alex and Jeff, who we met in Chapter 1, all compiled their portfolios in a conventional manner using folders and paper. However, it is likely that they all used computers to help them research, write, edit and store material before making their final selection. Increasingly, however, students are choosing to keep all their portfolio material in an electronic format. If this appeals to you, you will find Robbie's experience (described below) interesting. But do be sure to keep back-up files at every stage.

Case study: Robbie

Robbie, a first-year student, has collected a wealth of learning materials and competency assessments as evidence of his achievements. Unlike Aimee, Alex and Jeff, he has decided to keep his portfolio materials in an electronic form on his personal digital assistant (PDA). As a mature student, Robbie has had previous experience of using computers and could see the value of choosing an e-portfolio format as an effective and accessible way to showcase examples of his learning materials and competence assessments. Robbie was able to include multimedia elements from websites and CD-ROMS and DVDs as supplementary evidence of learning activities. In preparation for his first progression point meeting, Robbie organised all learning materials, mentor assessments and comments in the relevant sections of his e-portfolio. He found that the electronic format overcame logistical problems relating to showing his portfolio to his mentor and his personal tutor, and provided easy access for the external examiner as all his work could easily be downloaded to a memory stick.

Robbie says:

It was helpful to be able to view my work at the same time as my personal tutor, as this enabled immediate feedback and exchange of ideas. The computer facilities and sessions with the IT lecturers helped me to learn new skills. Eventually, after a very short time I found the e-portfolio easy to use and I became more proficient at filing records and materials in the right sections. My mentors also found using my PDA, while we were out and about working with different clients and agencies, useful to keep track of how much I was learning. A particular advantage was in being able to record our reflective discussions on my mobile phone and then uploading them later in the day. It helped me to remember what my mentor and I planned for the next week to develop my learning. I was also able to link in some material from one of the patient voice websites which had echoed my experience of working with particular clients. Now I wouldn't use any other way of keeping my portfolio other than electronically.

Robbie continues his story, reviewing the NMC Standards for mental health on p66 and describing the benefits of using his e-portfolio in community placements in Chapter 5 (p75). Meanwhile, Natasha (who you met in Chapter 1) has found herself increasingly using electronic media in connection with her portfolio. As a mature student, Natasha has a lot of experience of electronic file management from her previous career, and she has found this very useful for organising her competence assessment materials. She has also found that spreadsheets work very well when she is writing care pathways. She has brought good skills for searching for evidence on the internet with her into nursing, and this has enabled her to underpin her clinical skills experience with sound information. For a reminder of the merits of using e-portfolios versus paper-based formats, see Chapter 1 (pp13–14).

Linking NMC learning outcomes, domains, and generic and field competencies to your portfolio

A nurse's work is complex and often specialised. Many people have tried to define it, yet no one statement will suit all specialities and situations. Refer back to Activity 4.1 and review your findings of what people think a nurse does. The NMC consulted widely to gain agreement about what nurses should learn and be assessed in before they can enter the professional nursing register. The outcome of the consultation is a set of standards and competencies about what nurses should be able to do (NMC, 2010c). This is not a measure for the expert nurse, rather it gives a benchmark for a minimum acceptable level of competence to enter the NMC professional register.

Generic and field competencies

As you saw in Chapter 1, NMC generic and field-specific competencies are organised within four domains or categories:

- professional values;
- communication and interpersonal skills;
- nursing practice and decision making;
- leadership, management and team working.

The four domains listed above relate to each field of practice, namely adult, children's, mental health and learning disabilities nursing. Generic competencies represent knowledge, skills, attitudes and technical abilities required by nurses. Field-specific competencies relate to knowledge, skills, attitudes and technical abilities you must acquire in your specific field of practice. The number of field-specific competencies will vary in each domain and between fields of practice, and will increase over time throughout your programme. The field standards for competence make explicit the focus of approach for each specific type of nursing. The following NMC field standards for competence clearly show some similarities and some differences between each area of work.

> ***Adult nurses*** *must also be able at all times to promote the rights, choices and wishes of all adults and, where appropriate, children and young people, paying particular attention to equality, diversity and the needs of an ageing population. They must be able to work in partnership to address people's needs in all healthcare settings.* (NMC, 2010c, p13)

> ***Children's nurses*** *must understand their role as an advocate for children, young people and their families, and work in partnership with them. They must deliver child and family-centred care; empower children and young people to express their views and preferences; and maintain and recognise their rights and best interests.* (p40)

Learning disabilities nurses *must promote the individuality, independence, rights, choice and social inclusion of people with learning disabilities, and highlight their strengths and abilities at all times while encouraging others do the same. They must facilitate the active participation of families and carers.* (p31)

Mental health nurses *must work with people of all ages using values-based mental health frameworks. They must use different methods of engaging people and work in a way that promotes positive relationships focused on social inclusion, human rights and recovery, that is, a person's ability to live a self- directed life, with or without symptoms, that they believe is meaningful and satisfying.* (p22)

Essential skills clusters

Essential skills clusters (ESCs) do not include all the skills you will require as a qualified nurse but support the achievement of competencies and criteria for assessment at identified points in your programme. ESCs are for guidance and will be incorporated in your programme learning outcomes. There are five ESCs, as follows:

- care, compassion and communication;
- organisational aspects of care;
- infection control/prevention;
- nutrition/fluid management;
- medicines management.

Nurses completing the adult field of practice are required to meet the EU Directive (2005/36/EC), which relates to fitness to practise standards recognised across the European Union. Robbie's programme does not relate to the EU Directive because he is a mental health student.

Programme progression points to present your portfolio

You will achieve your learning outcomes, generic and field-specific competencies and ESCs in a range of settings. By periodically reviewing your portfolio your personal teacher and mentor can assess your progress in meeting NMC learning outcomes and competencies. There are likely to be two progression points, dividing your programme into three parts. Progress in acquiring competencies can be demonstrated by your achievement of minimum progression criteria based on safety and values which must be met in order to progress from one part of your programme to the next. Your first progression point will probably be at the end of Year 1, by which time you will need to demonstrate that you can be more independent in your learning and practice. The progression points will be an opportunity to showcase your learning achievements at a formal review meeting to demonstrate competency using the evidence you collected in your portfolio. (Refer back to the valid list of evidence shown earlier to demonstrate competence.)

Case study

Robbie reviewed the NMC Standards *for his mental health programme.*

I discovered the NMC generic and field-specific competencies also include essential skills clusters (ESCs). The standards, competencies and essential skills set out requirements which address what I must do and achieve during my programme and before I can become registered by the NMC. I looked at the ESC for care, communication and compassion for my second progression point and found I will need to develop appropriate and constructive professional relationships with family and other carers. This work will fit well with the ESC I have completed in Year I about building constructive relationships.

Activity 4.3	*Critical thinking*

1. In preparation for your next module, review a sample of generic and field-specific competencies for one module and write a short summary of how you will demonstrate achievement of competence.
2. Write a short summary of the ESCs that relate to one module and how you will demonstrate competence. Insert the summaries into the relevant sections of your portfolio.

You may wish to discuss what you have written with a friend or colleague who has completed the same exercise.

By the end of his first year Robbie had collected a wealth of learning materials and competency assessments as evidence of his achievements. You can find out more about these by turning to p75.

Conclusion

In this chapter we have argued that achievement of the NMC *Standards* and competencies can be demonstrated through an effective portfolio. We have also explored how a portfolio can be used to showcase evidence of learning activities in preparation for progression meetings. The extracts from Robbie's portfolio show how an e-portfolio can be an effective way to keep your evidence of learning.

The next chapter will go on to discuss changes in the learning environment and diversity of clinical placements. We will look at the plethora of learning resources, materials and people involved in your learning experience, and give helpful tips about using your portfolio across hospital and community settings. Examples of different scenarios will be given, including excerpts from patient stories and patient journeys. The differences between hospital and community learning opportunities will be explained.

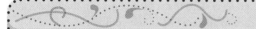

Chapter summary

First, this chapter has introduced you to the idea of using your portfolio to demonstrate competence. Second, you have been given some examples of how to identify valid work samples which can be used to demonstrate your competence. A link is included for your portfolio with NMC *Standards* and generic and field competencies. Tips have been given on how to prepare for progression point meetings with your personal tutor, mentor and possibly an external examiner. You have also been introduced to the idea of an increasingly popular approach to keeping portfolios, the e-portfolio.

Further reading

Benner, PE (1982) in Shobe, T, Nursing Expertise. *American Journal of Nursing*, 82 (30): 402–7.

Shobe describes how Benner's concern was not how to do nursing but how nurses learn to do nursing. She based her work on the Dreyfus model of skill acquisition, which she adapted to make it specific to the acquisition of skill where nurses pass through five levels of proficiency: novice, advanced beginner, competent, proficient and expert.

Directive 2005/36/EC of the European Parliament and of the Council of September 2005. *Official Journal of the European Union*, 30 September 2005, L255/22.

For nurses responsible for general care (adult), the Directive sets out the level, content and length of a programme. It facilitates nurses' mobility from one country to another within the EU and obliges member states to consider nursing qualifications acquired elsewhere in the EU to allow access to a regulated nursing profession.

Girot, EA (1993) The assessment of competence. *Nurse Education Today*, 25 (5): 355–62.

Girot concluded that nursing competency involved performing a task, knowledge of theory supporting the task and emotions a nurse possesses when carrying out the task. A holistic definition of competence is required because nursing requires a complex combination of knowledge, performance, skills and attitudes. The work has underpinned competency standards and clinical assessment tools.

Useful websites

http://standards.nmc-uk.org/Pages/Welcome.aspx

* *Standards for Pre-registration Nursing Education* (2010). These set out what nursing students must demonstrate to be fit for practice at the point of registration with the NMC. They contain the requirements and guidance that all approved institutions and their partners must adhere to in the development and delivery of education programmes.

- Field and generic competencies (2010). The challenges of the twenty-first century are much more complex and healthcare delivery is changing. Nurses of the future will practise differently. For example, adult and children's nurses will need to be able to care for people with mental health problems, while mental health and learning disabilities nurses will need to be able to care for people who have complex physical needs. The aim of generic and field-specific competencies is to ensure that when they graduate in their field of practice nurses will have high-level skills to care for people in their field, and also have knowledge and skills to provide essential care to anyone else in any setting..
- Essential skills clusters (2010). The ESCs are sets of skills which make up some of the learning outcomes and competencies in a programme. They must be met at certain progression points in a programme.

Chapter 5
Using your portfolio throughout your programme

> ### NMC Standards for Pre-registration Nursing Education
>
> This chapter will address the following competencies:
>
> **Domain 1: Professional values**
> 1. All nurses must practise with confidence according to *The Code: Standards of conduct, performance and ethics for nurses and midwives* (NMC, 2008), and within other recognised ethical and legal frameworks. They must be able to recognise and address ethical challenges relating to people's choices and decision making about their care, and act within the law to help them and their families and carers find acceptable solutions.
>
> **Domain 4: Leadership, management and team working**
> 7. All nurses must work effectively across professional and agency boundaries, actively involving and respecting others' contributions to integrated person-centred care. They must know when and how to communicate with and refer to other professionals and agencies in order to respect the choices of service users and others, promoting shared decision making, to deliver positive outcomes and to coordinate smooth, effective transition within and between services and agencies.

> ### Chapter aims
>
> After reading this chapter you will be able to:
>
> - identify the range and diversity of clinical placements available in hospital and community settings;
> - describe learning opportunities available in hospital and community settings;
> - create evidence to show a patient journey through the healthcare system including input from social services;
> - discuss ethical concerns about different levels of practice in hospital or community settings.

Introduction

Nurses have to deliver technical and skilled care across all health settings. The shift in emphasis towards a primary care-led service has profoundly affected traditional patterns of working, and the boundaries across healthcare professional roles and responsibilities are less clear. There is an increased overlap in knowledge, skills and attitudes between practitioners. The future challenges of healthcare will focus on long-term conditions, an ageing population and care outside hospitals. Effective care depends much more on each person's understanding of others' roles, and the need to work collaboratively within and between community and hospital teams.

Your placements will be planned to include time in community, hospital and other non-NHS settings so that you can develop an understanding of other health disciplines and multidisciplinary team working.

It is mandatory for students to complete annual manual handling, basic life support and fire prevention training. The verification of this training should be retained in your portfolio as it may need to be checked by your mentor.

In this chapter you will be introduced to Joanna, who is approaching the end of the second year of a pre-registration combined learning disabilities and social work programme. Joanna and Alex, our children's nurse from Chapter 1, share their experiences and challenges of working in a diverse range of placements across hospital and community settings.

Robbie, our mental health student, continues his story from Chapter 4 by describing the benefits of using an e-portfolio in community placements.

Making the most of your practice experience of the patient journey

More services are moving out of the traditional hospital setting and into the community and will be redesigned to deliver care closer to home. Nurses will therefore need to be competent to deliver care wherever service users access it. As in all placements, you will be supervised either directly or indirectly at all times. However, during the early part of your programme for experience in social care or in voluntary agencies you may be supervised by a suitably prepared registered professional who is not a nurse or midwife. In the final semester you will be supervised and assessed by a registered nurse. Some placements combine contrasting experiences in a range of hospital and community settings. You might be based in one environment but with short visits to another to observe different environments, commonly known as the hub and spoke model (see Appendix, pp111–14). Your mentor will use your portfolio as a communication tool to inform him/her of your overall progress. Practice placements are a vital part of your programme and experience must comprise at least 2,300 hours (50 per cent of the total number of hours) and there is an NMC requirement for practice placements for clinical experience to *be appropriate to meet NMC programme learning outcomes and for nurses to achieve field and generic competencies* (NMC, 2010c).

Figure 5.1 shows how one mentor identified a list of interesting learning opportunities for adult field students working in the community.

Mentor's advice on learning opportunities within a community placement

Here are a few people it will be helpful to spend some time with, in order to further your learning knowledge and understanding of interprofessional and multiagency care in the community (see competencies related to interprofessional working and multiagency collaboration in care). I have scheduled some of these opportunities into your timetable. However, you might like to follow a couple of patients over the next six weeks and make links to relevant services to understand holistic care.

- Coroner's court
- Community rehabilitation
- Carers' support service
- COPD nurses
- Community matrons
- Cardiac nurse specialist
- Heart failure nurses
- Diabetic nurse specialist
- Evening nurse
- Dermatology, wound care specialist
- Practice nurse

- Dietitian
- Midwife
- Social worker
- Falls prevention team
- Fast-track team
- H H day centre
- Hospice day centre
- Infection control
- Lymphoedema clinic
- Tissue viability
- Urology outreach
- Leg ulcer clinic

Please also see district nurse/practice teacher who organises fortnightly seminars for all students on community placements.

Evidence of learning can be submitted in several ways, e.g.:

- a patient pathway;
- a mind map showing understanding of different roles;
- visit notes;
- witness statement from relevant professional or agency.

Figure 5.1: Learning opportunities for adult field nursing students on placement in the community

If you are an adult nursing student you will have an additional requirement to meet the EU Directive (2005/36/EC) relating to experience in medical, surgical, maternity, mental health, children, older people and care in the home. You will be supernumerary to staff numbers until your final placement. An effective placement will enable you to:

- achieve NMC learning outcomes;
- identify learning opportunities;

- work alongside expert nurses and midwives;
- participate in activities which enable the application of theory to practice;
- learn about multiprofessional ways of working;
- observe and participate in care delivery;
- work within a team to learn collaborative approaches to care.

To give you an idea of the diversity and range of placement experience available, Alex (who we met in Chapter 1) and Joanne (who first appeared in Chapter 2) have listed below some examples of the acute and community placements they were allocated to for clinical experience. In each placement Joanne and Alex wrote a summary profile of their learning experiences to keep in their portfolio as evidence of key learning points and an insight into the focus of organisations and how they operate, and these are shown in Table 5.1, below.

Range and diversity of placements visited	Key learning points in organisations
Alex's learning in child care placements I visited another country for four weeks (funded visit to Spain)	I learned about the organisation and structures of children's nursing I experienced how resources are allocated in a different country
My experience of children's nursing in acute hospitals	I learned how sick children are cared for in an acute setting, including assessment, planning and evaluating their care and family-centred care
My learning about out-of-hours care of children in call centres, e.g. NHS Direct	I learned about government strategies and how parents of children can access health promotion and out-of-hours health advice I gained experience of telephone assessment and referral of children to GP on call or hospital for emergencies
My learning about children's nursing within multidisciplinary teams (MTD)	I gained knowledge of roles and responsibilities of the MTD to reduce fragmented care of children
Joanne's learning in learning disabilities placements I spent time in a residential care home	I learned about helping people with a learning disability with activities of daily living in a homely environment

Range and diversity of placements visited	Key learning points in organisations
My experience in nursing homes	I experienced caring for people with learning disabilities and with chronic and long-term conditions. Nursing homes provide the same level of care as in residential homes but with the addition of registered nurses who can deliver care for more complex needs. I learned about care standards and quality
My experience in the learning disabilities patients' own homes or of those who have difficulty accessing care in remote areas	I experienced care of learning disabilities patients in the comfort of their own homes in familiar surroundings, either before admission to hospital or living with a long-term or learning disability. This includes, for example, setting up equipment, teaching the patient or family members how to administer injections, or it might be for palliative care, wound care, etc.
Joanne and Alex: placements Our learning about nursing in the criminal justice system	We learned about legal and ethical frameworks for care in secure environments. We read about forensic procedures, Home Office and care protocols for high-risk learning disabilities patients and children who are a risk to themselves or others
Our experience of how out-patient nurses care for children and learning disabilities patients	They do not provide overnight hospital stay, so we learned about the importance of making sure the child/family/patient has support at home with an increase trend to performing more complex procedures
Where we learned about alternative types of healthcare	We spent a short time in the independent sector, private hospitals and specialist institutions such as those for children and people who have learning disabilities
We completed 300 hours of simulated learning	We were able to learn and rehearse skills in a safe environment using role play and problem-solving scenarios

(Continued)

Table 5.1 (Continued)

Range and diversity of placements visited	Key learning points in organisations
Our learning how voluntary agencies supplement community care	We experienced local services and voluntary agencies who often work in partnership with the NHS and other organisations. We learned how they offer assistance and advice to various groups of people such as carers of people with families
Our experience of learning nursing in residential schools. A minority of children with learning disabilities are cared for in residential settings	We learned how many of the children are in educational settings for much of their childhood. Input is provided by educational and social services

Table 5.1: Examples of Alex's and Joanne's diversity of placements and key learning points

---

Activity 5.1   *Critical thinking*

Select three or four placements from Joanne's list above and make a note of the kind of learning activities you could expect to find in relation to achieving the specific competencies listed. Refer to your module outcomes to remind you of the focus of your practice experience.

Compare your list with the information about learning opportunities given a little later in this chapter (p76).

Using your portfolio effectively across different settings

Undertaking experience in another country and (or) in placements across hospital and community settings means that you will have to keep a comprehensive record of your progress and learning achievements in your portfolio. This record is essential to provide continuity and effective communication between your mentors, your personal teacher, link lecturers and practice educators, who all will have an interest in your progression. Your assessment feedback across different periods of practice will need to be collated and shared between all of those involved in supporting and assessing you. Your consent must be sought to share any confidential information in your portfolio, such as a personal life/illness history that might influence your attendance, or dyslexia, with other people. You do not have to disclose these things but you may decide to in order to get specific and additional help. The NMC requires the following.

An on-going achievement record to be passed from one mentor to the next so that the student's progress can be judged. The student's consent should be obtained to share confidential data between successive mentors and education providers.

(NMC, 2010c)

As it will include your OAR and your clinical assessment document, your portfolio will be an important tool in presenting an ongoing overall picture of your learning achievements and maintaining continuity of practical assessments in a wide range of environments. Some community placements can be a distance away from your home base and you may be the only student. This would be unusual as universities try to pair students up when allocating them to a placement. If you experience problems, it is important to discuss your anxieties with your mentor, manager of the placement, link teacher or personal tutor.

Robbie, who we met in Chapter 4, found his format of choice a real bonus both for keeping comprehensive records and for working in a range of locations. By the end of his first year he had collected a wealth of learning materials and competency assessments as evidence of his achievements. In addition, Robbie was able to include multimedia elements from websites and CD-ROMS and DVDs as supplementary evidence of learning activities. (As discussed in Chapter 1, a paper-based portfolio can also be used to house the same materials if you have opted for this as an alternative.) In preparation for his first progression point meeting, Robbie organised all learning materials, mentor assessments and comments in the relevant sections of his e-portfolio. He found that the electronic format overcame logistical problems relating to showing his portfolio to his mentor, his personal tutor and the external examiner. Sometimes he found it helpful to be able to view his work at the same time as his personal tutor, as this enabled immediate feedback and exchange of ideas. At times, however, Robbie found that excessive and disorganised information in electronic form made him feel overwhelmed, so it is important to back up all your work and keep copies in relevant sections and categories of your portfolio.

Case study: Robbie's experience of using his e-portfolio in community placements

As a large number of my placements were in community settings, my e-portfolio allowed me to access and record work in any location. When I was in some of my longer community placements, I really valued the timetabled sessions I had with my tutor. In these sessions we could view my portfolio together and she would give me feedback with suggestions to make improvements. At times when I felt a little isolated I could ask for an extra session to be built in, which made me feel less remote. Eventually, I began to get more creative and customised my portfolio to my style, including my own care pathways from when I cared for a patient under the supervision of my mentor. Always I kept in mind the importance of the level of commitment and timelines when my work would be reviewed at the identified progression points in my programme.

Maximising your opportunities for learning

During your orientation/induction in each placement your mentor will usually identify which learning opportunities match your competencies. There are learning opportunities to achieve your NMC generic and field-specific competencies wherever nurses practise in hospital and community settings, and you should view every day and every placement as a potential for new learning. In the broadest sense, learning activities may relate, for example, to care approaches, care pathways or health promotion.

While 40 per cent of your time will be spent with dedicated support from a mentor, you will need to identify the other resources available to you. Examples include the MTD team, patients and carers as service users, patient support groups and other agencies that support clients.

Activity 5.2   *Reflection*

Write a comprehensive account of the roles, responsibilities and relationships of each team member for a team in which you have participated. Complete a mind map exercise to note your thoughts about the strengths and weaknesses of each role and how these impacted on care outcomes and decisions.

For an example of a mind map, see Samina's reflective mind map (Figure 2.3) on p36.

The patient's healthcare journey

It can be quite confusing to work out how separate organisations in the healthcare system fit together and how services are provided collaboratively by different agencies. Hopefully, the following information will provide you with an insight into a fairly typical patient's journey involving access across boundaries to provide what is described as a seamless service. You might think of a seamless service as smooth transition in delivering care activities between departments (see Figure 5.2). The healthcare system is made up of many different specialties, departments and offices. The first point of contact is the GP, who a patient will go to in the event of any problems or concerns. GP practices are often in groups or are linked together to share resources and expertise. The GP receives back results of any tests or investigations and will convey them to a patient. Any referral to the hospital for treatment is often made by the GP. Admission to an acute hospital is usually to complete further tests or to deliver medical treatment and care which cannot be provided in your patient's home. Acute hospital admission is a level of healthcare in which a patient is treated for a brief but severe episode of illness, for conditions that are the result of disease or trauma and during recovery from surgery. Acute care is generally provided by a variety of people using technical equipment and medication or medical supplies. The hospital stay will usually provide a diagnosis, nursing (multidisciplinary) care and medical treatment. In addition to providing critical care, the hospital will deliver a range of health and well-being services. There are different levels of help available for care in the home. Help which is outside personal care might include, for example, shopping, gardening or dog walking. Professional care at home or in their local community will generally help patients design and plan individual care packages that meet the needs of patients, families and the hospital requirements to ensure seamless transfer from hospital to home. Staff who deliver care in the home work to protocols and are CRB checked. Nurses and other multidisciplinary team members can provide education and training to patients and their relatives to enable greater independence, support and reassurance. The patient journey is a process which crosses organisational, primary and secondary care boundaries incorporating the patient's lived experience.

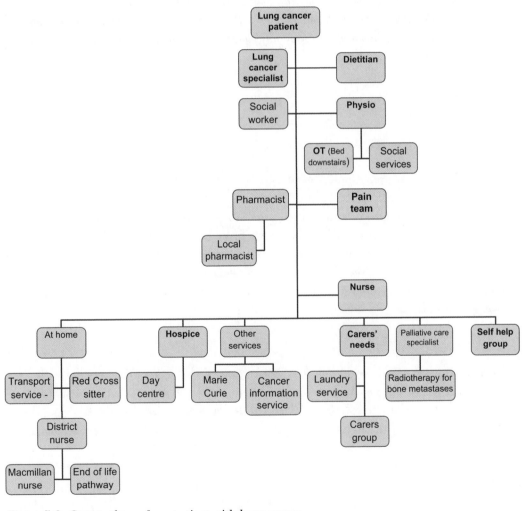

Figure 5.2: Care pathway for a patient with lung cancer

Activity 5.3 *Reflection*

Consider the typical patient healthcare journey outlined above and note the activities delivered by different departments.

Reflect on a patient you have cared for recently who has had a lengthy, complex journey. List some of the different personnel or departments this patient will have had dealings with. How do you think it might have felt to be passed from one to the other?

Case study

Joanne made an outline of a patient healthcare journey which involved primary care, a hospital stay and care provided in the home, for David, an adult with a learning disability who she had been visiting with a district nurse in one of her community placements. Joanne shares her outline example of David's healthcare journey below.

David's healthcare journey crossing organisational, professional and secondary care boundaries

PRIMARY CARE SUPPORT

David is a 40-year-old gentleman who lives at home with his elderly mother. David has mild learning disabilities and has also suffered from asthma since he was a child. The GP prescribes bronchial dilator medication for David. Although David's mother is fairly active, she gets tired easily when she tries to do too much and is unable to carry heavy shopping. Social Services provide support with home living for David and his mum, including shopping and meals. David enjoys meeting his friends at a club run by his social worker at which there is a weekly disco.

ADMISSION TO HOSPITAL

Having caught a heavy cold a few weeks before, David has developed a chest infection and is short of breath and wheezing. The GP visits David at home and decides to admit him to hospital. In the acute medical ward the doctor has prescribed nebulisers and oxygen therapy. Within a few days David is up and about, and is able to return home.

HOME CARE

David's GP has arranged for him to be visited daily by the community learning disabilities nurse to teach him to administer his inhalers correctly. Social services

continued ...

continued ...

have arranged meals on wheels to be delivered daily and for care assistants to help with bathing David's mum each week. An occupational therapist has completed a home assessment and arranged for hand-rails to be fitted around the house to help David's mum keep safe when she is moving about the house.

An information system between primary and acute care is important to reduce the risk of patients falling through the net, for example in GP referrals, patient discharge and out-patient follow-up. In record keeping, centralised patient records are helpful for multidisciplinary documentation to reduce the risk of misinformation, lack of information and duplication. The skills and knowledge Joanna has described in this chapter were all important for her development. She recorded her learning from them and her reflections, and inserted them into her portfolio along with assessments and feedback from her mentors.

Activity 5.4   *Critical thinking*

Using the healthcare journey example, describe the journey of a patient whose care you have been involved with. Follow the patient journey through the health and social care system. For example, start with primary care, involve a hospital admission, follow with care in the home and include input from social services.

Remember to insert your account of learning from this activity, and a note of how it links to a patient healthcare pathway, in your portfolio.

Activity 5.5   *Critical thinking*

Using the same healthcare journey example, refer back to the matrix of the 6Cs in Chapter 1 (pp11–12). Consider the physical, psychological and social needs of your patient and their family, and draw up your own matrix of behaviours and values which would be important in delivering high-quality care. Describe how each of the behaviours and values would be important in providing compassionate care.

Insert your matrix and description of behaviours and values in your portfolio.

Local and national governance frameworks

In hospital and community settings you could refer to clinical governance policies and procedures, and annotate how legislation affects your practice. For instance, risk-management policies will demonstrate the approach to identification and minimisation of risk to ensure public safety. It is important that you are aware of local clinical governance policies and procedures, and copies can be inserted in your portfolio to demonstrate your learning. You can be expected to be guided through a comprehensive induction in each placement, which usually will include aspects of local governance and risk management. All nurses and midwives have a professional duty to put the interests of people in their care first and to act to protect them if you consider they may be at risk. This applies to those people you know about or encounter during clinical experience, not just those people to whom you participate in delivering specific care.

Sometimes a patient's relatives are the first people to witness poor care. This was the case at a Staffordshire NHS hospital where complaints resulted in a detailed inquiry which examined the causes of failings in care standards and unnecessary deaths (Francis, 2013). Among wide-ranging aspects of the patient experience and a variety of care issues, nursing and nurse education were brought under scrutiny. Serious failures were identified, including not listening sufficiently to patients and staff; a tolerance of poor standards; and a disengagement from managerial and leadership responsibilities (particularly in nursing). Following the inquiry, a total of 290 recommendations were identified as necessary to bring about essential care improvements and changes throughout the entire healthcare system. One key change was identified concerning local and external reviews of safety and quality standards. The change relates to a shift in focus when accidents, errors and incidents occur. Previously, reviews would examine what went wrong to result in an accident, incident or error before identifying solutions and prevention measures. The new focus recommended by Francis (2013) is more about everyone being aware of what and how things should be done and then demonstrating commitment to ensure actions are evident in a prompt and timely manner. An additional recommendation in the Francis Report (Francis, 2013) refers to a legal duty of candour. The Nursing and Midwifery Council has called on nurses to tell patients when something goes wrong with their treatment or care, and have pledged to put openness and honesty at the heart of nursing (Merrifield, 2014). Actively listening to people's views and obtaining feedback from patients and relatives about the care they received is now considered paramount and has become a crucial aspect of every nurse's work. A common culture shared by all in the health service of putting patients first and all those who provide care to be made accountable for what they do are essential aims. Another important outcome of the Francis Inquiry is that students should not be placed for their practice experience in environments where patient safety is not adequately covered.

As a student, NMC principles and guidance are applicable to you and are underpinned by NMC *Guidance on Professional Conduct for Nursing and Midwifery Students* (NMC, 2009). It is important that you know how to raise concerns in any instances you believe service users are at risk or you observe poor quality of care, and there will be a whistleblowing policy to keep in your portfolio. It is recognised in the NMC publication *Raising and Escalating Concerns: Guidance for nurses and midwives* (NMC, 2010b) that it would not be easy for you to raise a concern about care or abuse. You may be unsure what to do or the process may seem daunting. You should inform your tutor, lecturer or mentor immediately if you believe that a colleague or someone else may be putting a patient at risk of harm. You should also seek help from your mentor, tutor or lecturer if people indicate that they are unhappy about their care or treatment. You might prefer to speak to your trade union or professional body if you are raising a concern, or you are worried generally about an issue, wrongdoing or risk which affects you, a patient or member of staff. You are acting as a witness to what you have observed or to risks that have been reported to you, and are taking steps to draw attention to the situation which could adversely affect those in your care, staff or the organisation. You should keep a record of the issues in your reflective diary and insert it in your portfolio as, in the event of future problems, you might need to recall events.

In some of the placements you may be required to wear appropriate protective clothing and this would be a good time to summarise reasons for special clothing in your portfolio.

Activity 5.6 — *Research and evidence-based practice*

Look at *The Code: Professional Standards for Practice and Behaviour for Nurses and Midwives* (NMC, 2015). How confident are you that you know what kind of behaviour is expected of you in a professional context?

Now visit the NMC website www.nmc-uk.org and go into the section on 'Hearings'. Read the FAQs on 'Fitness to Practise'.

Your Trust or employing authority should have a whistleblowing policy in place. Make sure that you are familiar with this and keep a copy in your profile.

Using the internet, look at a range of similar policies from different organisations, to see whether (and how far) they differ.

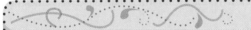

Chapter summary

In this chapter we have outlined care priorities of the future which have impacted on the need for you to be able to work in any setting in which service users access care. The importance of effective multiprofessional working and collaborative care is shown as the rationale for your experience in a diverse range of clinical placements. The variety of learning opportunities available wherever you are placed was described. Local and national frameworks were discussed in relation to governance policies and procedures which might impact on incidents and events in your placements. Chapter 6 will introduce you to assessment.

Further reading

Department of Health (2012) *Compassion in Practice: Nursing, Midwifery and Care Staff: Our vision and strategy.* London: HMSO.

The nursing strategy document setting out the shared purpose of nurses, midwives and care staff to deliver high-quality, compassionate care, and to achieve excellent health and well-being outcomes. It introduces the 6Cs.

European Union (2010) *EU Directive 2005/36/EC. Standards For Pre-Registration Nursing.* London: NMC.

Gives an account of cross-boundary working and team working. Augmentation of skills for nurses who work in hospital and in the community.

Francis, R (2013) *Report of the Mid Staffordshire NHS Foundation Trust Public Inquiry: Executive Summary.* London: Stationery Office.

Provides an account of the causes of failings in care and unnecessary deaths in the Mid Staffordshire NHS Foundation Trust.

Merrifield N (2014) NMC urges registrants to admit all errors in bid for openness. *Nursing Times,* 22 October, 10 (43).

An article from the *Nursing Times* describing how the NMC is attempting to instil a culture of openness and a candid approach to errors.

Nursing and Midwifery Council (2010) *Raising and Escalating Concerns: Guidance for nurses and midwives.* London: NMC.

Principles and guidance for student nurses about how to raise concerns and about whistleblowing procedures and policies.

Nursing and Midwifery Council (2010) *Standards for Pre-Registration Nursing Education.* London: NMC.

Discussion on the future roles of nurses and how working across boundaries and in collaboration will be key to delivering effective care.

Useful websites

www.institute.nhs.uk
A focus on the efficacy of the whole patient journey and how it is more important than the team's efficiency.

www.isdscotland.org/isd/3409.html
Typical NHS care and treatment in acute hospitals is described with definitions of emergency and severe illness.

www.nmc-uk.org
Full account of the *Standards for Pre-registration Nursing Education* (2010).

Chapter 6
Your portfolio and assessment

Chapter aims

After reading this chapter, you will be able to:

- describe the purpose and use of your practice competency assessments;
- identify what is used as the basis for making effective judgements about your clinical performance;
- be aware of what types of method are used to complete your practice assessments;
- identify who is accountable for determining your level of clinical competence;
- discuss the first and second progression points in your programme;
- show how your portfolio contributes to assessment.

Introduction

Your programme will equip you to meet present and future challenges in healthcare and to work in a range of roles providing complex care using the best available evidence and technology. Future services are likely to be delivered outside of hospitals. In each clinical placement you will be assigned a mentor who will be responsible for your achievement of learning outcomes. Mentors are formally prepared for their role by the completion of an NMC approved programme. They must have their name entered on a local register and are required to attend an annual update, ensuring they are up to date and current in practice. In the first year of your programme your assessor may not necessarily be a nurse and may not be on the same part of the NMC register as you. Final decisions during the last 12 weeks of your programme about whether you have achieved the required standard of competence for safe and effective practice for entry to the register must be made by a sign-off mentor. A sign-off mentor has completed formal preparation and also met additional criteria with identification on the local register and attends a triennial review as well as the annual update to keep familiar with your programme outcomes and documents. Clinical facilitators and link teachers provide support to mentors in completing your assessments.

In this chapter you will be introduced to Matthew, who is at the end of the second year of his adult nursing programme.

Six 'W' questions for the assessment of your portfolio

You might think of the assessment of your portfolio in terms of the six 'W' questions listed below. The questions have been adapted from steps frequently used in strategic planning.

- Why do your assessments need to be completed?
- What is it that is assessed?
- Which methods are used to complete your assessments?
- Who does the assessing?
- When will your assessments be completed?
- What form will feedback on your performance take?

A brief description of each of the above six 'W' questions is provided below.

Why: the purpose of your portfolio assessment

The NMC sets out the standard you must achieve to be deemed fit for practice at the point of registration. Standard 8 relates to outcomes, competencies and proficiencies assessed using a variety of assessment methods. All NMC outcomes in your programme are assessed as both written and clinical activities with each given equal weighting in your award. In the previous chapters you will have seen how your portfolio can collate:

- patient-focused assignments;
- reflective pieces;
- projects;
- care studies and care plans;

- clinical competence assessments or direct observation of your performance by an assessor;
- preparation for, learning from and results of your objective structured clinical examinations (OSCEs);
- constructive feedback from others;
- self-assessments.

Competencies are usually completed by an assessor or sign-off mentor directly observing a student performing a skill or number of skills in either simulation or in a real clinical setting. Assessments are either formative or summative. Formative assessment is not usually included in the formal grading of your evidence as it is developmental and can constitute a learning experience in its own right. An example of this might be writing an essay or a reflective piece, which are valuable activities for enhancing knowledge and skills. In contrast, summative assessment of your portfolio will usually generate a grade or pass/fail result of your evidence. Summative assessment is most often placed on completion of a piece of learning, module or programme denoting achievement. Formative assessment is ongoing, revealing your growth and development, leading to a first or second progression point, or finally at the end of your programme.

Activity 6.1   *Critical thinking*

Describe how formative assessment of a piece of work from an earlier module helped in the development of your knowledge and skills and application to practice.

Find an activity identified as summative assessment from any part of your programme. Compare the differences between the two approaches.

What: the basis for making assessment judgements and decisions about your evidence

The assessment of theory and practice is a continuous process with the standards for competence addressing knowledge, skills, attitudes, values and technical abilities that you must acquire to enter the NMC register. There are four sets of competencies, one for each field of practice: adult, mental health, learning disabilities and children's nursing. Each set comprises both generic and field-specific competencies. Generic competencies must be achieved by all nurses and field competencies relate to specific areas of practice. The number of field-specific competencies contained in each domain and between different fields of practice varies. The competencies are organised into four groups of activities called domains (NMC, 2010c):

- professional values;
- communication and interpersonal skills;
- nursing practice and decision making;
- leadership, management and team working.

Activity 6.2   *Reflection*

Look at your programme outline and your practice documents – how do they reflect the four domains for your programme? Identify the sets of generic and field-specific competencies contained in each for your field of practice.

Case study

Matthew is undertaking the adult nursing programme so he is required to complete EU Directives as set out in 2005/36/EC v2 {5.2.1} for general care in addition to field-specific and generic competencies. The adult nursing programme involves (evidence of) the assessment of theory and practice in a variety of settings. The range of settings where assessments will take place includes hospital, ward, clinic, patients' own homes, health centres and the community. There will be direct links between what is assessed in academic settings and what is assessed in practice, with both carrying equal weight. The theoretical and practice evidence you have gathered in your portfolio will be interpreted and assessed to make judgements about your competence. The whole process is overseen by an external examiner.

As Matthew is at progression point 2 and entering the final year of his programme, he will have already been confirmed as having met all requirements for his first progression point. He will be expected to become increasingly independent and encouraged to make decisions under the supervision of his mentor. He will need to demonstrate a high level of initiative and be able to put forward ideas to improve services and enhance patient care. Matthew will also be able to identify his own learning needs and plans and arrange the relevant practice learning experience and meet these needs as discussed previously in Chapter 1.

Matthew reviewed the NMC's essential skills clusters (2010a, 2010c) for his programme and found that ESCs include skills for the following groups:

- *skills for care;*
- *compassion;*
- *communication;*
- *organisation;*
- *infection control and prevention;*
- *nutrition and fluid management;*
- *medicines management.*

Which: methods used to complete your practice assessments

A variety of assessment methods will be used to test your acquisition of NMC learning outcomes and competencies. Performance assessment can be based on various types of simulation or on actual situations you are likely to come across that correspond to the NMC generic and field-specific competencies (NMC, 2010c). Competent does not mean expert. Education experts have devised several ways of assessing or illustrating stages of competency development. Your programme will be based on one of these or a combination. Beginners are rarely expert but they can be competent and can be distinguished from someone who is not a nurse or a student. You may find that you work slowly and are somewhat limited in the range of skills you can perform, but as you become more experienced you will gain confidence and will become increasingly efficient in completing tasks.

A variety of published rating scales are available and each university selects one that is suitable for your programme and to judge the level of competence you have reached. One way to assess

Stage 1: Novice	Student has no experience of the clinical situation in which he or she is expected to perform. Works in a 'just tell me what to do and I will do it' frame of mind.
Stage 2: Advanced beginner	Student can demonstrate an acceptable performance. Student has coped with real situations or has had them pointed out by a mentor. Performance is based on experience of a similar situation.
Stage 3: Competent	Typifies a student who has been in similar situations for 2–3 years. Sees actions in terms of long-range goals or future plans. Conscious, deliberate planning to achieve efficiency and organisation. Lacks the speed and flexibility of a proficient nurse.
Stage 4: Proficient	Perceives situations as a whole rather than chopped-up bits. Learns from past experience. Recognises when the expected does not materialise. Decision making is less laboured. Holistic understanding of the situation.
Stage 5: Expert	No longer has to rely on guidelines and rules to connect to the situation. Enormous background of experience of similar situations. Intuitive grasp of the situation. Does not waste time on trying to find other alternatives. Knows when the action looks right and feels right. Has a deep understanding of the total situation.

Table 6.1: Five stages of clinical competence

(Source: based on the work of Benner, 1982)

performance is to measure expected behaviours that are anchored as statements or dimensions of a skill, ranging from competent to incompetent. The statements reflect a group of competencies called domains. One example is the Benner (1982) five-point novice to expert scale (referred to briefly earlier in Chapter 4), which places a student at a particular point on the scale according to how their performance of a skill best matches specific criteria. Level 3 is noted as competent. The Benner stages of clinical competence are shown in Table 6.1.

An alternative scale to Benner's novice to expert scale is the Bondy (1983) performance rating scale, which is commonly used in nursing education assessments. Criteria define and explain student behaviours and activities that are matched to a level of performance of NMC field-specific and generic competencies when observed by an assessor. The clear demarcation points also identify those students who need help and further development. The fair assessment of performance provides a mentor/assessor the means of giving valid and reliable diagnostic feedback. Matthew proved achievement of his competencies by presenting summaries of his learning and his clinical competence assessments in his portfolio. Each mentor that Matthew was allocated to wrote comments and feedback statements about his progression in his portfolio. Matthew has provided an example of his competence in patient assessment using the Bondy rating scale below. You will see that level 3 is similar to the NMC definition of progression point 1 at the end of Year 1 of the pre-registration nursing education programme. Matthew placed himself at Bondy level 4, which identifies him as being at the end of Year 2 (progression point 2). Progression point 3 at the final stage of the programme is similar to Bondy's independent level 5.

Label	Score	Quality	Level
Bondy dependent level 1: A beginning student. Matthew is mainly observing his mentor when she is completing a patient assessment.	Student is unsafe, inaccurate, unskilled.	Student is unable to perform patient assessment due to lack of insight.	Assessor statement: *Matthew requires continuous physical direction and verbal cues by his mentor to complete patient assessment.*
Bondy marginal level 2: A student at the early stages of learning. Matthew participates in patient assessment under supervision of his mentor.	Student is not completely accurate; unskilled, inefficient.	Student is safe only with guidance.	Assessor statement: *Matthew requires frequent physical direction and continuous verbal cues in patient assessment.*

Label	Score	Quality	Level
Bondy assisted level 3: Similar to NMC progression point 1 – end of first year. Matthew participates under the supervision of his mentor to complete a patient assessment.	Matthew is safe and accurate and has achieved some NMC competencies, including NMC safeguarding of people of all ages/ carers/families.	Matthew is proficient throughout some of the activities for completing a patient assessment, including NMC professional values and attitudes towards people, carers, families.	Assessor statement: *when completing a patient assessment Matthew requires frequent supportive verbal cues.*
Bondy supervised level 4: Matthew has reviewed the NMC clinical competencies for patient assessment and, confirmed by his sign-off mentor, has placed himself at Bondy level 4. Matthew is at progression point 2 at the end of his second year.	Comments noted by Matthew's mentor fit with Bondy level 4 – *Matthew is safe, accurate and has achieved NMC competencies for completing a patient assessment. Matthew is also reasonably efficient.* Matthew's sign-off mentor has verified that *Matthew is able to communicate effectively with people in vulnerable situations.*	Matthew's mentor has written a statement noting: *Matthew is reasonably confident.* Matthew's sign-off mentor has verified that *Matthew is more independent with patient assessment and he ensures dignity is maintained at all times.*	Matthew's mentor stated: *he requires occasional verbal cues in patient assessment.* Matthew's sign-off mentor has verified that *Matthew requires less supervision in patient assessment. Also, Matthew takes more responsibility for his learning and practice.*
Bondy independent level 5: Similar to NMC progression point 3 – final part of the programme.	Matthew's sign-off mentor states: *Matthew is safe and accurate and has achieved all NMC competencies related to patient assessment.*	Matthew's sign-off mentor has verified: *Matthew is proficient, confident and efficient in all competencies related to patient assessment.*	Assessor statement: *Matthew does not require any cues or prompts to complete a full patient assessment.*

Table 6.2: Assessing Matthew's level of competence using the Bondy (1983) performance rating scale

After a period of formative development and observation a mentor or sign-off mentor will draw conclusions about your competence and produce a summative evaluation of your clinical ability and performance.

When asked about their understanding of competencies, students often describe eight different activities, listed below (Ramritu and Barnard, 2001), which they see as essential to being a nurse:

- safe practice;
- limited independence;
- utilisation of resources;
- management of time and workload;
- ethical practice;
- performance of clinical skills;
- knowledge;
- evolving care within the scope of professional practice.

Interestingly, the list proposed by the students in 2001 indicated performance of skills as essential to being a nurse. However, clinical competence did not feature in the activities. Seven years later, Bradshaw and Merriman (2008) examined how nurses are prepared to be clinically competent and safe at registration, so they are fit for practice and purpose. The study focused on whether nurses acquire certain specific clinical skills. The introduction of clinical skills laboratories, objective structured clinical examinations, clinical assessments, self-assessment and simulation of practice has resulted in a variety of clinical assessment techniques. The study concluded there is no uniform system in place to ensure all nurses are clinically competent and safe to practise.

Activity 6.3   *Critical thinking*

Refer to Benner's (1982) five stages of clinical competence, the Bondy (1983) rating scale for performance measurement criteria and the eight activities of a competent nurse described by newly qualified nurses above. Compare the criteria provided by each of the rating scales and the eight activities of a competent nurse and consider what is your understanding of what it means to be a nurse and how good is good enough to be called a competent nurse.

Both Benner and Bondy have included five levels of performance in their rating scales. Other rating scales available are smaller and provide only two options from which to select a level of performance. Some universities prefer to use, for example, a simple pass or fail grading system, which denotes that the student has achieved learning outcomes or requires further development.

Activity 6.4	*Group working*

In a small group of, say, four to six other students from your cohorts, match the levels 1–5 in the above rating scales (or one you are more familiar with) to either the generic or the field-specific competencies from a clinical placement experience you have completed. Discuss the criteria for expected behaviours and share your views on how closely you each match the expected behaviour. Identify where each of you fits in terms of needing more direction or supportive cues or supervision. Use the grid provided by Matthew, from his assessment document below, for you and your colleagues to record your competence level in patient admission.

Matthew has provided an example of one skill from his assessment document to help you to complete Activity 6.5 on p92.

Matthew's example of NMC generic and field-specific competencies for the adult nursing programme and assessed levels of competence

NMC 2010 Competencies for adult nursing

Domain 1: Professional values
Generic standard for competence

All nurses must act first and foremost to care for and safeguard the public. They must practise autonomously and be responsible and accountable for safe, compassionate, person-centred, evidence-based nursing that respects and maintains dignity and human rights. They must show professionalism and integrity, and work within recognised professional, ethical and legal frameworks. They must work in partnership with other health and social care professionals and agencies, service users, their carers and families in all settings, including the community, ensuring that decisions about care are shared.

Level of competence achieved: identify with an asterisk which level is appropriate (refer to the description of levels provided by Benner and Bondy).

level 1   level 2   level 3   level 4   level 5

      **

Signature of mentor/sign-off mentor: ———————————————————————

Signature of student: ———————————————————————————————

Date achieved: ————————————————————————————————

At progression point 1 (at the end of his first year) Matthew's sign-off mentor had identified him as level 3 for the generic competency standard for adult nursing, which is defined in the Bondy performance rating scale as *assisted, safe and accurate, achieved most competencies, proficient throughout most of performance when assisted, requires occasional physical direction and frequent verbal cues.*

Field standard for competence

End of Year 2

All nurses must support and promote the health, well-being, rights and dignity of people, groups, communities and populations. These include people whose lives are affected by ill health, disability, ageing, death and dying. Nurses must understand how these activities influence public health.

Level of competence achieved: identify with an asterisk which level is appropriate (refer to Bondy's description of levels).

level 1   level 2   level 3   level 4   level 5

                 **

Signature of mentor/sign-off mentor: ————————————————————

Signature of student: ————————————————————

Date achieved: ————————————————————

By progression point 2, Matthew's sign-off mentor had identified him as Bondy level 4 for the field-specific competency example level of assessment but Matthew will need to get to Bondy level 5, which is independent, by progression point 3 at the end of Year 3. All competency assessments and the ongoing achievement record will provide a sound base for final, overall judgements and decisions about fitness to enter the NMC professional register.

Activity 6.5   *Reflection*

Compare one field-specific and the generic competency identified above by Matthew with those for your own programme, and note what level of competence described by Bondy or Benner is appropriate for you at this point in your programme.

Who: makes judgements and decisions about your level of competence?

The NMC *Standards* require that you be assessed in a range of settings such as hospital wards and departments, the community, patients' homes and health centres using a variety of assessment methods. Assessors may be NHS or non-NHS, health practitioners who complete your NMC assessments and non-health practitioners who provide informal feedback. Service users are increasingly becoming part of the assessment process. Examples of service user involvement in assessment include:

- providing views on care delivered by a student;
- participation in OSCEs;
- participation in assessment, planning and evaluation of care;
- practitioners and employers providing views about student fitness for practice at the end of a programme and their employability possibilities.

In some parts of your programme you may be required to complete a self-evaluation. Self-evaluation and self-assessment are used interchangeably and are terms used to define a process by which you rate the quality of your own work and critically review your own performance. Self-assessment is usually completed by referring to criteria set out in a performance rating scale similar to the examples provided on pages 87–9 by Bondy and Benner. Other tools you could use include, for example, a simple pass or fail grade or asking a colleague: 'how am I doing?'

When: the progression points in your programme

As programmes prepare students for a career in nursing and also for life-long learning opportunities the NMC has identified two progression points which separate your programme into three equal parts. Practice assessment is a continuous process, which means that a mentor will be observing your performance at all times in your placements. There are progression points identified by the NMC to provide distinct stages for confirming that a student is able to continue on the programme or may require further focused help and development. Normally, a student would be identified as needing development to meet learning outcomes before a progression point occurs. Your progress in acquiring competence is based on meeting safety and values criteria through the use of minimum progression criteria. The criteria are based on safety and values which you must meet in order to progress from one part of your programme to the next. The first progression point is at the end of your first year and the second is at the end of the second year. Then progression point 3 is at the final part of the programme. Some examples of NMC criteria for progression have been linked to levels of working and supervision in Table 6.2 on p89 with the Bondy rating scale. NMC essential skills clusters have not been identified for all progression points and they do not include all skills and behaviours needed of a qualified nurse. They are incorporated into your learning outcomes and assessments throughout your programme, but after the second progression point and before entry to the register they should be achieved in full. Remember how Mike decided to leave his assessment on drug administration until his third year because he wanted lots of practice (see p30)? You may also prefer to defer some competency assessments until you feel confident.

In Table 6.3 Matthew provides an example of a competency about safeguarding adults and children to show his development and increasing independence from his first progression point up to the final part of his programme.

First progression point End of Year 1	Second progression point End of Year 2	Third progression point End of Year 3
Acts within legal framework and local policies in relation to safeguarding adults and children who are in vulnerable situations. Evidence example – statement by mentor in clinical assessment document: *is aware of appropriate behaviour and Trust policies in relation to safeguarding adults and children.*	Documents concerns about people who are in vulnerable situations and at risk or in need of support and protection. Evidence example – confirmation by mentor that competency achieved in relation to *good documentation and comprehensive and accurate record keeping in relation to concerns about people who are at risk or in need of support and protection.* Countersigned by a qualified nurse.	Recognises and responds when in vulnerable situations and at risk or in need of support and protection. Evidence example – confirmation by sign-off mentor of achievement of competency about *recognition and response when people are in vulnerable situations and at risk or in need of support and protection.*

Table 6.3: Matthew's progression points and evidence of achievement of safeguarding competence

---

Activity 6.6   *Decision making*

Consider your first or next progression point. What do you need to prepare for the meeting with your mentor, personal teacher and link lecturer? Make a note of all of the assessed evidence you have collated in your portfolio to demonstrate your level of competence.

What: the form that feedback on your practice assessments should take

Your ongoing achievement record (OAR) is part of your practice assessments and will move with you from one placement to the next to assist your mentors in judging your progress. Universities usually provide two types of document for practice assessments. The OAR document specifically targets any development areas identified in previous placements so that your mentor can focus on highlighted learning needs. The continuous assessment document sets out the NMC generic and field-specific competencies and essential skills to be achieved and often also includes a professional conduct section. The document will provide sections for your mentor to:

- make comments about your performance;
- report your progress and development;
- highlight any concerns requiring attention and future monitoring;
- indicate actions to address your individual learning needs;
- indicate actions and agreements to address any concerns about attitude and behaviour;
- indicate the minimum level of performance you have achieved;
- add their signature to verify that you have achieved NMC learning outcomes, generic and field-specific competencies or essential skills.

Not all placements will require you to complete a summative assessment; some learning experiences will be formative with a log of learning activities signed by your mentor to keep in your portfolio as a record. Because the OAR contains important details about your level of competence and behaviour, you will be asked for your consent to share any confidential data between successive mentors and sign-off mentors.

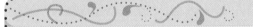

Chapter summary

The discussion in this penultimate chapter should help you to understand the importance of your portfolio in assessment. Looking back over this chapter, you will be able to take away key points about the why, what, how, who and when of how your portfolio is included in assessments. In some programmes the portfolio acts as the base for assessment. You should also have an insight into the form that the feedback you receive will take. It is a good idea to actively pursue feedback from others by getting into the habit of asking them their views on how you are progressing and how you might improve.

The final chapter in this book will provide you with an insight into the way you can use your portfolio throughout your career and how it will equip you to prepare for important job interviews and appraisals.

Further reading

Benner, PE (1982) In Shobe, T, Nursing expertise. *American Journal of Nursing*, 82 (30): 402–7.

Provides a detailed description of criteria by which to judge a level of performance a nurse has reached. Shows the five stages of development from novice to expert and all stages in between.

Bondy, K (1983) Five-point rating scale. *Journal of Advanced Nursing Education,* 22 (9): 376–82.

A comprehensive description of the five-point rating scale used in performance assessment. Provides a detailed explanation of criteria used to decide the level of student competence.

Bradshaw, A and Merriman, C (2008*)* Nursing competence 10 years on: fit for practice and purpose yet? *Journal of Clinical Nursing,* 17 (10): 1263–9.

Describes the changes to nurse education in the UK and lack of uniformity in clinical assessments.

Chapter 7
Your career and your portfolio

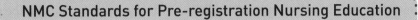
Chapter aims

After reading this chapter you will be able to:

- prepare to enter the NMC register;
- describe using your portfolio as part of self-regulation;
- be aware of the NMC requirements for revalidation;
- put together a career plan;
- describe the benefits of your portfolio as part of an employment interview;
- describe using your portfolio as part of your appraisal once you are qualified;
- discuss the value of your portfolio for marketing yourself for future job prospects.

Introduction

Preparation to enter the NMC professional nursing register

Entering nursing means accepting accountability for practice and being up to date. It is a legal requirement to hold appropriate cover under an indemnity arrangement. Should you opt for a post in an NHS setting you will already have this under their procedures. However, if you work in areas other than the NHS you will need to make your own professional indemnity cover arrangements. It is crucial that your portfolio is refined as you prepare for registration with the NMC. The national nursing strategy for England emphasises the importance of reconnecting staff to the values and behaviours that underpin their work to keep compassion at the heart of how care is delivered (DH, 2012). You will need to demonstrate through your portfolio that you have stayed connected to the 6Cs (discussed in earlier chapters) and how you establish core working principles to align your organisation's goals to your own individual ones. Your portfolio is not just something that you discard when you complete your final assessment and join the nursing register: it is something that you should continue to refine and maintain as your nursing career develops and will be a valuable tool when you go through the revalidation process every three years.

This chapter will introduce you to Maggie, who has recently completed her pre-registration mental health nursing programme. Maggie shares her experiences of the use and benefits of her portfolio for working with her preceptor to identify strengths and weaknesses for effective support and development. Maggie provides some useful tips for career planning and her first employer interview. Eventually, your portfolio will help in preparing for your first appraisal. The importance of showcasing your abilities and accomplishments is covered, and Maggie gives some examples of how she has successfully marketed herself in her career through effective use of her portfolio. Also included in this chapter are some tips from Rachel, the adult nursing student from Chapter 3, who shares her experience on how to set goals for realising professional aspirations.

How to put together your nursing career plan

Once you have achieved registration as a nurse with the NMC for a specific field of practice, you will need to decide how to continue to develop your career. Some options to choose from might be, for example:

- working in clinical practice;
- teaching nursing students;
- involvement in research in clinical practice.

Activity 7.1   *Reflection*

Take a good look at who you are and consider your personality and your career aspirations.

Reflect on the following questions and make a note of your thoughts.

- What type of nursing (refer to the list above) do you want to do?
- What are your main nursing interests (e.g. working with acutely ill patients, emergency departments, older people, people with long-term conditions, etc.)?
- What are your key strengths (e.g. dealing with people who have hearing or sight deficits; responding quickly in emergency situations, etc.)?

continued ...

---

continued ...

- What are your professional values (e.g. maintaining dignity of people, compassion, caring, etc.)?
- What are your main assets and attributes (e.g. calm in emergency situations, good at working in a team, good at decision making, etc.)?
- What are your passions and ideals (e.g. high-quality care, value for money, etc.)?
- What would be your ideal workplace environment (e.g. a busy place, a calm and peaceful place, working in the community, etc.)?
- What are your favoured skills sets (e.g. pre-operative preparation, patient admission, nutrition, infection control, etc.)?

Maben et al. (2010) believe that when newly qualified nurses enter the workforce their values, ideals and compassion are clearly evident. Seedhouse (2012) stated that nurses enter the profession with a sense of altruism, but as training progresses they become less empathic and more distant from patients. Burnout, stress and unsupportive working conditions can lead to cynicism or complacency developing over time and you may find that some of the more satisfying aspects of the nursing role can be lost as you become increasingly taken away from care delivery to fulfil other commitments such as administrative duties. Taking the time to regularly reflect on your values and remind yourself of why you have entered nursing will be important to ensure you continue to deliver compassionate and empathic care.

Maggie has agreed to share her five-year plan for her career in mental health nursing (see Table 7.1).

My nursing career goal	To become a specialist nurse practitioner in mental health
My current nursing skills and knowledge	Registration with the NMC as a nurse (mental health)
My short-term career goals	Obtain a job for experience as a staff nurse for one year on a mental health in-patient unit. Supported by preceptor
Ongoing professional development	Complete mentorship programme. Become a sign-off mentor and enter local register. Complete annual updates and triennial review
Long-term career goals	Work as a specialist practitioner (mental health) for two years
Ongoing professional development	Complete nurse prescribing programme to prescribe in mental health

Table 7.1: Maggie's mental health nursing career plan example

Activity 7.2	*Decision making*

Make a plan of your intended career. This could show where you would like to be in your career in five years' time. You will need to show the path to achieving promotions for your dream jobs and what type of experience and qualifications you will need to progress on your career ladder. Streamline your portfolio, discarding any documents that do not add to your professional credibility and make you shine. Present all documents so that materials are well organised, secure and in order. Add your career plan to your portfolio.

Preparing for your first job interview

An interview is the most crucial part of the recruitment process. Your portfolio will include a massive amount of evidence from your pre-registration programme, a lot of which might not be relevant to a job interview, so you definitely will need to discard some of the materials.

How will you match the job description and fit into your chosen workplace?

You will need to regularly update all materials in your portfolio to truly reflect your skills and attributes. Each time your portfolio is used for a new job you will need to focus the materials to make it fit for purpose and specific to the post applied for. You will need to be very selective about what evidence to include and what to discard to demonstrate your high level of credibility and match yourself to the job description and specification. Generic examples of what could be relevant to any job interview might include:

- experience and acquisition of skills sets in relation to the job description;
- project/research experience, especially highlighting any skills that might transfer to requirements of the post;
- clinical activities and acquisition of NMC generic and field-specific competencies for the field of practice you would prefer to work in;
- critical analysis and reflective excerpts from experiences you had as a student to demonstrate you are able to use the skills for care improvements;
- reports, care studies, care pathways and care plans to demonstrate your ability to write clearly, concisely and accurately;
- acquisition of knowledge to underpin your professional practice to demonstrate effective decisions and judgements based on sound, up-to-date evidence;
- mandatory training certificates such as manual handling, resuscitation, fire training and infection control;
- completion of any voluntary work and highlighting any skills or experience as evidence of team work.

Your portfolio linked to job applications

Competition for nursing jobs is getting harder all the time so your portfolio will need to stand out from all the other applicants. If two people are being interviewed for the same job, then the person showing most enthusiasm, motivation and interest will most likely be the one who will advance in future vacancies that might come up in the organisation. Your portfolio will need to do the following.

- Provide a résumé or concise curriculum vitae; this will be a separate section in your portfolio and will include clear, concise statements about you. What is important to you in your career? What professional values and ideals do you hold about nursing? Someone, somewhere could be looking for someone just like you, so highlight the attributes and strengths you have. What are your future aims? What goals do you want to achieve?

- Be specific; make a good impression about your achievements. Know something about the place and the people by searching websites because this may provide a few pointers to what kind of workplace it is and the type of person they are looking for. Indicate that you have read current relevant policies and reports.

- Be focused on the key points of the job specification; go through each point and look on the website at the organisation's mission statement. Show your intention to grow into new positions in due course and to better your knowledge and skills through the experience of the job you have applied for.

- Be comprehensive and remember that less is more; showcase your accomplishments, especially in relation to the desired job.

- Have you been a course representative? What did you learn from the experience? What skills and knowledge did you gain, for example did you act as a voice for others and negotiate changes to your programme?

- Include complimentary and positive feedback and comments from your mentors.

- Include certificates, diplomas and qualifications to confirm your competence.

- Include academic staff positive feedback comments on your marked assignments.

- Include cards and letters from patients or staff – show things you are proud of.

- Include personal references with names, addresses, telephone numbers and job titles of the referees (these should not be relatives).

Activity 7.3   *Research and evidence-based practice*

Review the job specification and job description for the post you have applied for. Make a note of key words and cross-check with materials in your portfolio to see where you match the requirements of the post. Produce a CV and a smaller, customised portfolio for a specific job interview and be prepared to be ruthlessly selective over what is included. Put your best achievements at the forefront. Ask a friend or colleague to look through what you have in place and maybe make suggestions for any clarification required. Retain any discarded materials elsewhere as they may be required at another time for a different purpose.

How a potential employer might use your portfolio

Your potential employer will probably ask to view your CV, so it's important that key points about you are on the front page. They may ask to review your portfolio before or after the interview. Then, if you are successful, they may wish to see it at various stages as it is valuable in showing your strengths and weaknesses and your transition through the first year in your new post. Any weaknesses or gaps will be highlighted, so your employer will be able to help you address them through guidance and support or developmental training and **preceptorship**.

When you start your new job you will not have the back-up of your tutors, so do not hesitate to ask questions as people will usually appreciate your willingness to admit that you do not know everything. It is important to get the balance right as you should not appear over-anxious, under-confident or needy.

Activity 7.4	Reflection

Refer back to your personal development plan from Chapter 1: use the template and start afresh, or you might just wish to update and develop it. This will show you as a person who can plan goals and set targets to achieve your aspirations.

Using your portfolio in your first appraisal

Appraisal is a way of evaluating your current and future performance in your role and to indirectly improve the quality of care you deliver to patients. The appraisal will also help you and your employer to ensure you are supported and developed in your role as an employee. All individuals have different needs and their capacities vary, so the appraisal provides an excellent opportunity for:

- setting future career and role performance action plans, the means to set target achievement dates and a process of continual development;
- clarifying your employer's expectations of you and increasing your motivation;
- clarifying your expectations and aspirations to your employer about where you aim to be in, say, five years' time;
- reinforcing where any further development is needed, for example if you want to develop towards a future leadership post;
- reinforcing good achievements, raising standards for quality care, recognising accomplishments and how well you are doing; acknowledging your contribution, making you feel valued and giving you a sense of belonging;

- setting the foundation for a good working relationship between you and your employer, and thereby providing benefits to both;
- initiating any changes that need to happen.

How to prepare for your appraisal

The appraisal is usually an annual (or more often) occurrence in most organisations. However, the annual event should be preceded by informal dialogue, discussion and meetings throughout the year. This will allow time for improvement of any weaknesses highlighted before the actual appraisal event. People generally can become quite nervous about the impending scheduled date of the event. The appraisal is not in any way a platform for disciplinary actions; it is non-judgemental and a formal process comprising forms, checklists, interviews, discussion, objective setting and action planning. However, on rare occasions, if you are not achieving all that is expected, an action plan may be put in place together with supervision and monitoring.

How to get the best out of the appraisal meeting

The event will be arranged well beforehand with time set aside to reinforce the importance, as a priority, of the appraisal system. It is unusual for an appraisal to be cancelled unless in exceptional circumstances. Often there is a self-evaluation component to give you an opportunity to reflect on where you are now and where you next want to be on the career ladder. You might feel a little uncomfortable about evaluating yourself and rating your own performance, but it is important to be realistic otherwise it makes it difficult for your employer to inform you of their perceptions which might differ from yours.

Top tips for getting the most out of your appraisal

- Prepare all year round by collating relevant materials in your portfolio.
- Write reflections on your achievements and keep them in your portfolio.
- Speak up about your accomplishments in any informal meetings with your boss.
- Listen carefully to what others tell you about how you are doing in your job.
- Take the positive and the negative comments as constructive and helpful for your development.
- Be open and receptive to advice from experts who have been there in the same situation themselves.

Following the interview and discussion, it is usual to agree objectives with your employer to make explicit your targets and aims. An action plan with the process for achievement completes the appraisal event.

How to put together your action plan

Your manager will have been trained in completing appraisals and will set you aims, objectives and future plans together with dates for achievement and review of the progress you have made. In Chapter 2 we looked at setting action plans using the SMART process. It is equally valuable in appraisal.

Setting SMART objectives

SMART objectives are commonly used in evaluating and appraising performance whereby targets are set for employees who must fulfil the criteria. SMART is an acronym for writing goals and targets which will meet the requirement for future review and measurement. Doran (1981) provided a set of key and minor terms which explain the meanings of each letter in the acronym.

Key definition	Associated definitions
Specific	Significant, simple
Measurable	Meaningful, motivational, manageable
Attainable	Appropriate, achievable, agreed, actionable, aspiration-aligned, ambitious, assignable
Realistic	Do not under-set the bar; not too stretched; resourced
Timely	Time-framed, time-based, tangible, time-tabled, time-specific

Table 7.2: Terms and definitions for the SMART acronym (Doran, 1981)

Maggie was fortunate to be offered the first post she applied for: a staff nurse post on an in-patient psychiatric ward. Maggie has been allocated a preceptor who will oversee her work and provide support and clinical supervision for the first four months of work. Maggie has agreed some SMART objectives with her preceptor for the first four months and she has agreed to share an example.

> ### Case study: Example of Maggie's SMART objectives
>
> Specific: I would like to be proficient in the care of 3/4 different patients who have depressive illness symptoms.
>
> Measurable: I will demonstrate the effective care of 3/4 patients.
>
> Attainable: I will demonstrate the smooth, efficient and effective care of 3/4 patients who receive therapy for depressive illness.
>
> *continued ...*

continued ...

Realistic: I may care for only one patient who has depressive illness during the next three months.

Time-orientated: I will complete the above list in 3-4 months.

DUMB objectives

As an alternative to SMART objectives another acronym (DUMB) was used by Rachel's employer to set targets for her to achieve. DUMB objectives are used in strategic and business planning but can be applied as part of an action plan following an appraisal.

Case study: Explanation of Dreamy, Unrealistic, Motivating and Bold acronym used by Rachel

Dreamy

Goals that make you wonder if something is possible.

Rachel wrote: I would like to become a clinical manager in ITU in five years' time.

Unrealistic

Goals that traditionalists warn against, and believe are not attainable by anyone.

Rachel wrote: eventually I would like to be a member of the Trust Board or be a chief executive.

Motivating/manageable

Goals that mean you are ready to take on the day.

Rachel wrote: I am so looking forward to being team leader today and hope to be a good one.

Bold

Goals that chart a course that competitors do not dare to take because of fear of failure or because they find success too daunting.

Rachel wrote: I am confident I can complete the nurse prescribing programme to work towards my plan for working in clinical management. This development will benefit my employer by expanding the nurse prescribing workforce numbers. This development will also benefit my patients by providing them with access to my skills as a nurse prescriber.

Signature of employee: ———————————————

Date: ———————————————

Signature of appraiser: ———————————————

Date: ———————————————

Maggie has agreed to share her second appraisal form to help you to complete the next activity.

Case study: Example of Maggie's second appraisal form

Name of employee Maggie Fitzgerald	NMC PIN 6543210	Date of expiry June 2012	Qualifications RN (MH)

Study days attended in last year

Clinical Governance Issues and Policies.

Mandatory training you attended in last year

Fire training, manual handling, cardiopulmonary resuscitation.

Mentor update date; triennial review dates

Completed January 2011; due 2012 (arranged).

What are your main achievements in the last year?

I successfully completed the Mentor Training Programme. My name has been entered on the local Trust mentor register.

My Practice Education Facilitator has arranged the triennial review dates for me to retain active mentorship on local register.

What challenges did you encounter resulting in you not achieving your objectives?

Did not develop intended knowledge and skills in risk management.

What key areas of work need to be covered in the coming year?

Prepare for Mentor Triennial Reviews. Develop risk management techniques.

What additional skills and knowledge do you need?

Specialist practitioner skills and knowledge. Develop knowledge and skills for evidence-based practice.

What additional training do you need?

Complete Specialist Practitioner Programme at degree level.

What other issues do you need to discuss?

Possible plans for reconfiguration of the mental health service and how they might affect me and my practice.

> ### Activity 7.5   *Decision making*
>
> Your employer will very likely provide you with a template for the type of appraisal form they wish you to complete. In preparation for your first appraisal interview apply the above example to your own situation adding your SMART or DUMB goals.

Using your portfolio to market yourself

Your portfolio might also be valuable to help you to advance on the career ladder or for a job change. If you are looking for a career change you might decide to enlist the services of a nursing recruitment agency that will search for suitable job vacancies which could be of interest to you. The agency may well use your portfolio to market your skills with a potential employer, so it is crucial that it is clear and professionally presented to make a good impression, and dividers and page protectors should be inserted. Make a few duplicate copies of your portfolio. Write an introductory page and summary leading into the materials to follow. As well as including examples from the above list in your portfolio you might consider including:

- any specialist skills and knowledge you have developed;
- any conferences you have attended that show you are forward thinking and current in your practice;
- any workshops you have attended such as risk management, clinical governance or health and safety;
- any publications you have participated in writing or have written yourself;
- any awards or honours you have received;
- a picture of yourself (optional).

Many post-registration programmes require completion of a portfolio as part of the assessment strategy. In addition, you could submit an accreditation portfolio to be awarded exemption from certain aspects of a programme. This is called APEL or accredited prior experiential learning, which means being awarded credit for learning outcomes already achieved. Your portfolio would need to show a close match to meeting criteria in the programme. You may eventually decide to pursue a career as an advanced practitioner and it is possible that your portfolio could provide part of the application and selection process to gain a place on the programme as well as a base to build on for assessment purposes.

How to remain on the NMC professional nursing register

In response to the Francis Inquiry Report (2013) the NMC has developed a revised model of revalidation. The failings identified by Francis were extremely serious and the NMC instigated wholesale changes to the way that registered nurses are audited. The new system was designed to protect the public more effectively and ensure that all nurses remain fit to practise across their entire career. Nurses are now required to regularly provide evidence that they are up to date and still able to deliver high standards of care. This is vital if the public are expected to trust the nursing profession. The new revalidation process (see www.nmc-uk.org/revalidation) represents a stringent audit that you will need to pass every three years in order to remain on the register. It is closely linked to the NMC *Code* (2015) and designed to be a crucial means of reinforcing professionalism.

When revalidating, every nurse and midwife will be required to confirm that they:

- continue to remain fit to practise;
- have met the requirements for practice hours and continuing professional development;
- have sought and received third party feedback which has informed their reflection on their practice; this feedback could be from patients, carers, students (for educators) or peers;
- have sought and received third party confirmation that they are fit to practise. A third party (likely to be a manager, another registrant or a supervisor) will need to confirm that the nurse or midwife is adhering to the *Code* and *standards*, and is fit to practise.

The involvement of a third party is significant. For example, an employer or a manager will need to confirm that you have practised for 450 hours during the last three years, and the amount of continuing professional development (CPD) you have completed will be reviewed and clarified as suitable. In this way an extra level of scrutiny and supervision is added to the process with nurses now required to actively demonstrate and prove their commitment to CDP. There are many forms of CDP and it will be down to you to identify and judge what activities best demonstrate this, but there will be many instances where examples of high standards of practice could be corroborated by managers or employers. For instance, they could confirm that you have completed particular higher education or training, or verify that you have been on a secondment to broaden your practice experience and develop new skills.

At the time of writing, the new revalidation process is still being tested and finalised, so you are well advised to consult the NMC website (www.nmc-org-uk.org/revalidation) for the latest information. It is important to be aware that the work you do developing and maintaining your portfolio as a student nurse will provide you with valuable transferable skills and an ideal method for organising materials and evidence to show how you can meet the requirements of revalidation. The NMC (2014) currently recommends that you permanently maintain a portfolio between revalidations and use it as a basis for discussions with your third party confirmer (e.g. your line manager). The NMC may also ask to see your portfolio in order to verify the declarations you make when submitting your revalidation application. Examples of evidence you might provide include:

- administrative activities, providing clear and accurate records, care pathways and reports about patient care;
- teaching activities with other staff or with patients or relatives;
- involvement in research projects and participation in project management;

- supervised practice and development in management and leadership roles;

- direct patient care provision, application of the 6Cs to practice, audit and monitoring of clinical practice.

You should collate any materials and evidence relating to the above list and retain them in your portfolio. You will be responsible, and held accountable, for your own revalidation process and you must take active measures to maintain your competence through regular professional development.

The ongoing development of your portfolio as part of self-regulation

Each time you use your portfolio you will need to ensure you have presented your evidence in a clear, professional, organised format. A well-presented and comprehensive portfolio will provide an opportunity to organise your evidence in accordance with the NMC *Standards*. Your personal portfolio will by now include a great deal of evidence from your pre-registration programme showing a trail of materials to demonstrate your development and progression. Some of these materials from your pre-registration programme will include signatures and comments from your sign-off mentor(s) attesting to and verifying your competence and fitness for practice on a legitimate basis. Current NMC registration provides a licence to practise and is compulsory for anyone wishing to work as a nurse, midwife or health visitor in the UK. Your registration will provide proof that you are a qualified, competent person, and someone who is worthy of trust and confidence.

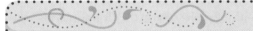

Chapter summary

The end of this chapter denotes the end of the book. Hopefully, you will have picked up some useful tips and be more aware of different approaches for compiling a successful portfolio. This chapter has focused on using your portfolio as part of NMC self-regulation and how, once you are on the register, you can maintain your registration. It has also looked at using a portfolio to help you prepare for a job interview and appraisal.

Further reading

Bauer, R (2011) SMART Goals are out DUMB Goals are in.

Available at: www.evancarmichael.com/Marketing/1160/SMART-Goals-are-out-DUMB-Goals-are-in.html.

An alternative approach to setting goals.

Department of Health (DH) (2012) *Compassion in practice* Leeds: Department of Health.

A strategy document setting out the shared purpose of nurses, midwives and care staff to deliver high-quality, compassionate care, and to achieve excellent health and well-being outcomes.

Doran, GT (1981) There is a S.M.A.R.T. way to write management's goals and objectives. *Management Review,* 70 (11): 35–6.

Provides a description of how to write SMART goals and full explanation of associated terms and definitions.

Francis, R (2013) *The Final Report of the Mid Staffordshire Foundation Trust Public Inquiry Executive Summary.* London: Stationery Office.

Maben, J, Cornwell, K and Sweeney, K (2010) In praise of compassion. *Journal of Research in Nursing,* 15 (1): 9–13.

Nursing and Midwifery Council (NMC) (2014) How to revalidate with the NMC (draft document). London: NMC.

Seedhouse, D (2012) Developing compassion in pre-registration nurse education. *Nursing Times,* 110 (37).

An article considering how to instil compassion into nurse education.

Standing, M (2014) *Clinical Judgement and Decision Making in Nursing* (2nd edition). London: SAGE Publications.

A nursing textbook introducing an evidence-based approach to clinical judgement and decision making. The final chapter introduces the 'PERSON' evaluation tool, which is a helpful framework for nurses to use when evaluating their clinical practice.

Useful websites

www.ehow.com/how_4896827_write-nursing-portfolio.html
Gives simple steps on putting a portfolio together for a job.

www.evancarmichael.com
A web link which provides discussion as an author blog with full explanation of DUMB goals and associated terms and definitions.

www.nmc-uk.org/Nurses-and-midwives/Revalidation/
Background information and guidance on the NMC revalidation process.

www.nmc-uk.org/Nurses-and-midwives/Revalidation/Revalidation-resources/
Resources elaborating on the new revalidation process.

www.nmc-uk.org/Registration/Professional-indemnity-arrangements/
Information on the professional indemnity arrangements for registration with the NMC.

Appendix
Suggested programme for potential placement experience for a student using the hub and spoke model

How the hub and spoke model works

Possible Insight visits
Family care team
– home visits
– coffee mornings
– safety training

Hearing screeners • Physio • Dietitian • Pharmacist • Theatres
Transport team • Crash bleep team • Labour suite
Pregnancy assessment clinic   Consultant follow-up clinics
– high-risk pregnancies   Postnatal wards
– diagnosis of abnormalities   – transitional care
– baby checks with SHO

SPOKE
Children's Medical Ward

SPOKE
Children's Development Centre

HUB
Placement
Name
Neonatal Intensive Care Unit

Directorate/Locality
Family Health

Suggested number of weeks 'at base' before first spoke
4–6

SPOKE
Paediatric Intensive Care/ High Dependency Unit

SPOKE
Children's Surgical Unit

SPOKE
Neonatal Surgical Unit

Third-year student (children's nursing) Neonatal intensive care unit, 27 weeks

Weeks 1–2: HUB Low-dependency area	Orientation to placement area Basic care of babies, e.g. temperature monitoring, nappy changing/skin care Different feeding methods Communication with parents Care planning/evaluation
Weeks 3–4: HUB High-dependency area	Care of sick/premature babies Intensive monitoring Communication with parents Care planning/evaluation

Week 5: INSIGHT

Postnatal wards – prenatal care of mums at high risk of preterm delivery, emotional care after delivery of preterm/sick baby, conditions in mums which may cause premature delivery

Labour suite – care of women in premature/high-risk labour

Pregnancy assessment/ultrasound – care in high-risk pregnancy, diagnosis of abnormalities

Crash bleep team – immediate resuscitation of preterm or sick baby

Transport team – transfer of sick or premature baby from DGH to intensive care

Weeks 6–9 HUB
High-dependency area

Weeks 10–11: SPOKE Paediatric high-dependency/intensive care units Caring for ex-neonatal patients, appreciation of ongoing care needs	**Weeks 12–13: SPOKE Neonatal surgical unit** Caring for babies with surgical conditions Theatres to observe surgical treatment

Week 14: INSIGHT Multidisciplinary team

Family care team – home visits, home oxygen, support of families

Hearing screeners

Dietitian – feeding supplementation, PN, importance of nutrition/growth

Physician – developmental care, assessment of development, positioning/exercises to support development

Pharmacist – improve medication knowledge

Baby checks with SHO – development of knowledge of normal and common abnormal findings in babies

Consultant follow-up clinics – ongoing care/development/support of babies post-discharge

Neonatal support groups/playgroups – what support is available, how families cope day to day

Weeks 15–16: SPOKE Children's general medical/general surgical ward	**Week 17: SPOKE Children's development centre**
Immediate ongoing care of babies discharged directly from neonatal to paediatric care with long-term problems	Specific clinics, e.g. neurodevelopment
Readmission of babies/children who have previously required neonatal care	Respite care of children with complex needs, knowledge of difficulties faced by babies discharged from neonatal care in later life

Weeks 17–18 HUB
Management – low-dependency area

Care planning, moving babies towards home

Parent teaching in preparation for discharge, e.g. bathing, feeding, temperature monitoring, medication administration, spotting illnesses, emergency care/resuscitation

Discharge planning meetings; liaison with other agencies, e.g. home oxygen, postnatal wards, outpatient clinics, medical staff, community midwife/health visiting teams, GPs, family care team, arranging TTOs/equipment for discharge

Managing team of other nurses and healthcare assistants to coordinate and prioritise care of all babies in low-dependency area

Weeks 19–27 HUB
Management – high-dependency area

Admission of sick babies, both preterm and full term, expected and unexpected intensive monitoring and treatment methods

Intensive care strategies, e.g. ventilation, cooling for HIE, blood gas analysis

Patient assessment and care planning

Recognising and managing deterioration

Resuscitation

Managing and prioritising a workload

MDT working: doctors, consultants, pharmacists, physios, dietitians, radiologists, surgeons

Parent support, dealing with anxiety, helping to encourage bonding and involvement of care in the baby

(Continued)

Staff allocation

Ward round

Managing staffing levels

Liaison with delivery suite, postnatal wards, transport team regarding admissions and available bed spaces

Arranging transfer to referral (e.g. surgical, cardiac units) or referring (e.g. DGH for continued care after intensive care) centres as appropriate

Glossary

Clinical governance A system of audit and other checks health services use to check on and improve their services.

Confidentiality Only divulging information that has been given by a patient to the people with whom the patient has agreed the information may be shared and not sharing the information beyond this group. It is a cornerstone of nursing practice.

Critical thinking Questioning one's own and others' assumptions, addressing gaps in knowledge to achieve aims, challenging illogical or unethical beliefs or practice, evaluating strength of available evidence, and the ability to present a logical, evidence-based argument and defend it when challenged.

Evidence Any kind of information that is used to support reasoning, problem solving, clinical judgement and decision making, including observations, feedback, policy, theory and research.

Learning style A preference for particular ways of learning.

Mentor A registered nurse who has met the requirements of the NMC mentorship standard and is responsible and accountable for facilitating learning and assessing competence of students in a practice setting.

Nursing Promoting health, prevention of or recovery from illness or injury, adaptation to disability, or dignity in facing death in patient-centred care by applying bio-psycho-social-spiritual knowledge, skills and ethical values to safe, effective judgement, decisions and evidence-based practice.

Ongoing achievement record (OAR) A document that provides evidence of the progression in practice of nursing students and demonstrates their achievements to successive placement mentors as they move from placement to placement and year to year.

Personal development plan (PDP) A framework and plan of action drawn up by students and qualified nurses identifying their own strengths and weaknesses, and including plans for building on the former and addressing the latter by additional learning. The PDP, which will be closely linked to the professional portfolio, will also outline some goals for a future path.

Preceptorship A period of practical experience, or 'training on the job' in which the student nurse is supervised by an expert in the field.

Reflection Considering and reviewing thinking, actions and circumstances to develop new ideas.

Reflection-in-action Knowing what to do in order to make a difference within a given situation.

Reflection-on-action Examining some of those 'in the moment' decisions for the possibility of other choices and ways of acting, and how these insights might shape and develop future practice.

Reflective practice Considering and reviewing the interplay between theory, practice and new ideas.

References

Bauer, R (2011) SMART Goals are out DUMB Goals are in. Available at: www.evancarmichael.com/Marketing/1160/SMART-Goals-are-out-DUMB-Goals-are-in.html (accessed February 2015).

Benner, PE (1982) in Shobe, T, Nursing expertise. *American Journal of Nursing*, 82 (30): 402–7.

Bondy, K (1983) Five-point rating scale. *Journal of Advanced Nursing Education*, 22 November, 9: 376–82.

Bradshaw, A and Merriman, C (2008) Nursing competence 10 years on: fit for practice and purpose yet? *Journal of Clinical Nursing*, 17 (10): 1263–9.

Clark, AC (2010a) How to compile a professional portfolio of practice 1: aims and learning outcomes. *Nursing Times*, 106 (41): 12–14.

Clark, AC (2010b) How to compile a professional portfolio of practice 2: structure and building evidence. *Nursing Times*, 106 (42): 14–18.

Clark, D (2008) Honey and Mumford's Learning Styles Questionnaire. Available at: www.nwlink.com/~donclark/ hrd/styles/honey_mumford.html (accessed February 2015).

Department of Health (DH) (2001) *What is a Portfolio?* London: HMSO.

Department of Health (DH) (2012) *Compassion in Practice*. London: HMSO.

Doran, GT (1981) There is a S.M.A.R.T. way to write management's goals and objectives. *Management Review*, 70 (11): 35–6.

European Parliament (2005) *Directive 2005/36/EC. Official Journal of the European Union*, 30 September, L255/22.

European Union (2010) *EU Directive 2005/36/EC: Standards For Pre-Registration Nursing*. London: NMC.

Finnerty, G, Volante, MA, Rockingham, L, MacLaren, L and O'Driscoll, M (2008) Promoting a deep approach to professional learning in the field. Development and evaluation of electronic personalised learning. Centre for Research in Nursing and Midwifery Education. Division of Health and Social Care, Faculty of Health and Medical Sciences, University of Surrey. Available at: www.surrey.ac.uk (accessed February 2015).

Fisher, A and Scriven, M (1997) *Critical Thinking: Its definition and assessment*. Norwich: University of East Anglia, Centre for Research in Critical Thinking.

Francis, R (2013) *Report of the Mid Staffordshire NHS Foundation Trust Public Inquiry: Executive summary*. London: Stationery Office.

Frankel, A (2009) Nurses' learning styles: promoting better integration of theory into practice. *Nursing Times*, 105 (2): 24–7.

Girot, EA (1993) The assessment of competence. *Nurse Education Today*, July 2005, 25 (5): 355–62.

Honey, P and Mumford, DA (2000) *The Learning Styles Helper's Guide*. Maidenhead: Peter Honey Publications.

Howatson-Jones, L (2013) *Reflective Practice in Nursing* (2nd edition). London: SAGE Publications.

Hutchfield, K (2010) *Information for Nursing Students*. Exeter: Learning Matters.

Kolb, DA (1984) *Experiential Learning: Experience as the source of learning and development*. Upper Saddle River, NJ: Prentice Hall.

Latham, D (2014) Test for nursing values unveiled. *Nursing Times*, 10 (3).

Lintern, S (2014) Prior experience for students is the bottom line. CNO Summit Lord Willis. *Nursing Times*, 110 (51).

Maben, J, Cornwell, J and Sweeney, K (2010) In praise of compassion. *Journal of Research in Nursing*, 15 (1): 9–13.

McMullan, M (2008) Using portfolios for clinical practice learning and assessment: the pre-registration nursing student's perspective. *Nurse Education Today*, 28 (7): 873–9.

Merrifield, N (2014) NMC urges registrants to admit all errors in bid for openness. *Nursing Times*, 22 October, 10 (43).

Mobbs, R (2003) Honey and Mumford learning styles. Available at: www.le.ac.uk/users/rjm1/etutor/resources/learningtheories/honeymumford.html (accessed February 2015).

National Quality Board/NHS England (2013) How to ensure the right people with the right skills are in the right place at the right time: a guide to nursing and midwifery and care staffing capacity and capability. Available at: www.england.nhs.uk/wp-content/uploads/2013/11/nqb-how-to-guid.pdf.

NICE (2013) *Safe Staffing for Nursing in Acute Hospitals.* London: National Institute for Health and Care Excellence.

Nursing and Midwifery Council (NMC) (2006, reissued with new cover 2010). *The PREP Handbook.* London: NMC.

Nursing and Midwifery Council (NMC) (2007a) *Guidance for the Introduction of the Essential Skills Clusters for Pre-registration Nursing Programmes.* London: NMC.

Nursing and Midwifery Council (NMC) (2007b) *Standards for Medicines Management.* London: NMC.

Nursing and Midwifery Council (NMC) (2008) *The Code: Standards of conduct, performance and ethics for nurses and midwives.* London: NMC.

Nursing and Midwifery Council (NMC) (2009) *Guidance on Professional Conduct for Nursing and Midwifery Students.* London: NMC.

Nursing and Midwifery Council (NMC) (2010a) Medicines management. In *Essential Skills Clusters and Guidance for Their Use* (guidance G7.1.5b). London: NMC, pp32–41.

Nursing and Midwifery Council (NMC) (2010b) *Raising and Escalating Concerns: Guidance for nurses and midwives.* London: NMC.

Nursing and Midwifery Council (NMC) (2010c) *Standards for Pre-Registration Nursing Education.* London: NMC.

Nursing and Midwifery Council (NMC) (2014) How to revalidate with the NMC (draft document). London: NMC.

Nursing and Midwifery Council (NMC) (2015) *The Code: Professional Standards for Practice and Behaviour for Nurses and Midwives.* London: NMC

Price, B and Harrington, A (2013) *Critical Thinking and Writing for Nursing Students* (2nd edition). London: SAGE Publications.

Quality Assurance Agency for Higher Education (2009) *Personal Development Planning: Guidance for institutional policy and practice in higher education.* Gloucester: QAA.

References

Ramritu, PL and Barnard, A (2001) Newly qualified graduates' understanding of competence. *Nursing Review*, 48 (1): 47–57. First published online, July 2008.

Read, C (2014) More work to do to make the 6Cs universal. Report of the CNO for England Summit 2014. *Nursing Times*. Special edition, 110 (50).

Scholes, J, Webb, C, Gray, M, Endacott, R, Miller, C, Jasper, M and McMullan, M (2004) Making portfolios work in practice. *Journal of Advanced Nursing*, 46 (6): 595–603.

Schön, D (1984) *The Reflective Practitioner. How professionals think in action*. London: Temple Smith.

Seedhouse, D (2012) Developing compassion in pre-registration nurse education. *Nursing Times*, 110 (37).

Strivens, J, Baume, D, Grant, S, Owen, C, Ward, R and Nicol, D (2009) The role of e-portfolios in formative and summative assessment: report of the JISC-funded study for recording achievement for JISC. Centre for Recording Achievements. Available at: www.jisc.org.uk (accessed February 2015).

Timmins, F and Dunne, PJ (2009) An exploration of the current use and benefit of nursing student portfolios. *Nurse Education Today*, 29 (3): 330–41.

University of Salford School of Nursing (2007) *Personal Development Planning Resources Pack*. Salford: University of Salford.

Watterson, L (2013) 6Cs + Principles = Care. *Nursing Standard*, 27 (46): 24–5.

Index

Page numbers in *italic* refer to figures and tables.

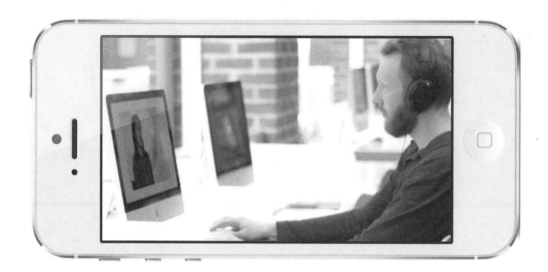

⑤SAGE video

We are delighted to announce the launch of a streaming video program at SAGE!

SAGE Video online collections are developed in partnership with leading academics, societies and practitioners, including many of SAGE's own authors and academic partners, to deliver cutting-edge pedagogical collections mapped to curricular needs.

Available alongside our book and reference collections on the *SAGE Knowledge* platform, content is delivered with critical online functionality designed to support scholarly use.

SAGE Video combines originally commissioned and produced material with licensed videos to provide a complete resource for students, faculty, and researchers.

NEW IN 2015!

- Counseling and Psychotherapy
- Education
- Media and Communication

sagepub.com/video
#sagevideo

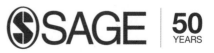